GRANNY gets a NEW KNEE

and a whole lot more

LOUISE CHEGWIDDEN

Illustrations *by* Mokhtar Paki

Text copyright © 2014 by Louise Chegwidden

Cover and internal illustrations copyright © 2013 by Mokhtar Paki

Gold Rush illustration copyright © 2013 by Julian Mayotte

All rights reserved. This book is protected by copyright. No part of this book may be reproduced in any form or by any electronic or mechanical means, including information storage and retrieval systems, without permission in writing from the publisher, except by a reviewer, who may quote brief passages in a review. Please purchase only authorized electronic editions, and do not participate in or encourage electronic piracy of copyrighted materials. Your support of the author's rights is appreciated. Any member of an educational institution wishing to photocopy part or all of the work for classroom use, or anthology, should send inquiries to the author: info@GrannyGetsANewKnee.com.

Printed in the United States of America

ISBN: 978-0-9915507-0-8

Book Design by Alvaro Villanueva

*"Movement is life. Life is a process.
Improve the quality of the process
and you improve the quality of life itself."*
—*Moshe Feldenkrais*

Dear Reader,

For seven years, the first draft of a book to help people get the most out of knee replacement surgery sat in a drawer under my computer. It was sound, but not appealing. Full of practical information, but lifeless.

Then Granny and Jerome wrote themselves into my life, bringing their humor, compassion, and inspiring eagerness for learning. They gave me a story that offers the same information woven into the larger context of their everyday lives.

The result is before you in two parts:

Part One: GRANNY GETS A NEW KNEE, written in dialogue form, follows Ms. Mattie (Granny) as she meets her movement teacher, Ms. Linda Thomas, attends classes, practices what she learns, and organizes her support team before and after knee surgery.

Part Two: AND A WHOLE LOT MORE includes the six movement lessons that Granny practices (plus one Just For Fun!), how to use them effectively, and other helpful information–all the written materials that Granny received from Ms. Linda.

My sincere hope is that with the assistance of this book, you find much more than relief from knee pain.

With great respect,
Louise Chegwidden
September 14, 2013

Contents

Introduction 11
Who's Who 12
It's Time. 13

PART ONE: GRANNY GETS A NEW KNEE
B.S. (BEFORE SURGERY)

Granny's Kitchen 14
First Class or Soft Shoe Shuffle. 15
Shoes 17
Second Class or Twist Again 21
A Special Note from Granny 24
Third Class or Helicopter Circles 26
Granny's First Acupuncture Visit – EVER! 29
Fourth Class or Climbing The Walls 31
Preparations 35
Fifth Class or First Movements 37
TLAs 43
Sixth Class or The Floor is My Friend 46
Lists And Logistics 48
Granny Goes in For Surgery 51

A.S. (AFTER SURGERY)

Sanchez Kitchen	53
Practice, Practice, Practice	55
Revolving Door	57
Practice Buddies	59
Breathing Up and Down	61
Delora's 'Back to School' Dinner	65
Snap	67
All the Way Up	69
First Outing	71
Granny's Walking Route	74
Happy Gardening	75

PART TWO: AND A WHOLE LOT MORE

Before You Start	78
Pain and Ice and Elevation	80
Notes To Helpers	81
Improving Movement = Reducing Unnecessary Effort	83
Scanning Your Contact	84

THE LESSONS:

- Lesson 1: Soft Shoe Shuffle Primer 86
- Lesson 2: Twist Again 88
- Lesson 3: Helicopter Circles 90
- Lesson 4: Climbing The Walls 92
- Lesson 5: First Movements 94

* Lesson 6: The Floor Is My Friend 96
* Just For Fun 99

SUGGESTED DAILY SCHEDULE AFTER SURGERY

In the Hospital 102
At Home 104

KEYS TO MAKING PROGRESS, SAFELY.

Keep Moving 106
Transitions 107

THE BIG PICTURE:

Breathing 110
The Two Elephants in the Room — Gravity and Time . . 111
Resting 111
Equipment List 112
Frequently Asked Questions 113

ABOUT MS. LINDA

Biography 117
The Feldenkrais Method of Somatic Education 117

PS

A Special Note from Ms. Louise 119
Without Whom … 120

Introduction

Hi.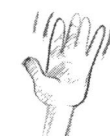

My name is Jerome Evan Sanchez, and I'm eleven years old.

This is the story of my Granny's new knee.

I'm writing it down so you can help someone in your family get the most out of their knee surgery too.

I hope you like my drawings.

(Look for this picture throughout the story to find 'Jerome's Notes')

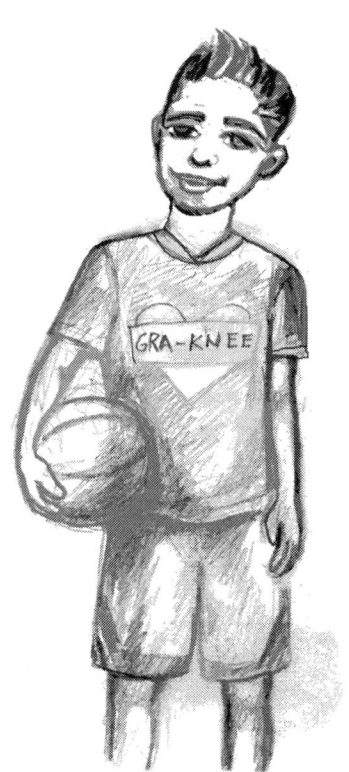

Who's Who

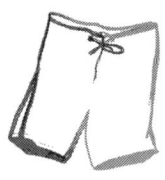 : That's me. Those are my favorite basketball shorts.

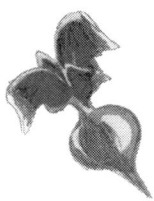 : That's Granny. She's the one in the family with a green thumb.

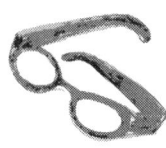 : That's my Mom, Deisha. She just got those glasses for reading.

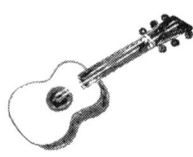 : That's my Dad, Ernesto. He loves his guitar.

 : That's my cousin Delora. She's a brainiac AND a college All State player.

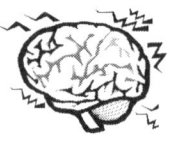 : That's Ms. Linda. She's putting the sense back in the Sensory-Motor System.

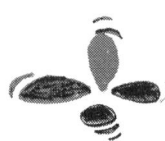 : That's an interesting sound.

It's Time

My Granny lives next door to me, and for the last six months, every Tuesday and Thursday, I help her. It's on account of her knee. She rubs it all the time, says she knows when it's going to rain, and has been taking too many pain pills. I hear that's not good for her kidneys.

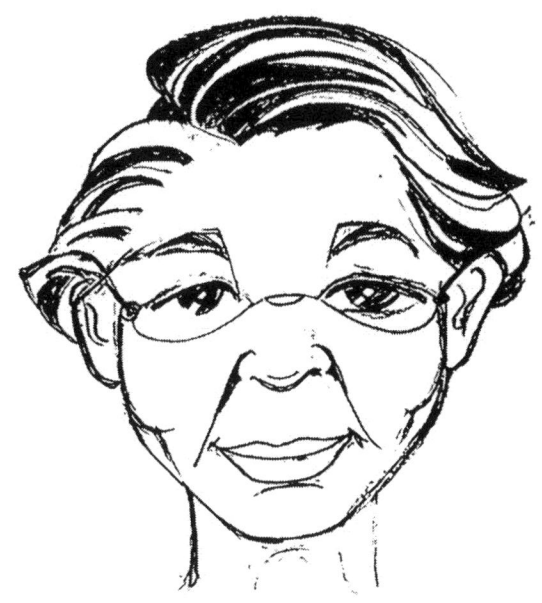

I think it's time for a new knee and her doctor agrees with me. But first, she has to get ready. She'll be going to some classes taught by a movement-learning specialist who is also a Physical Therapist. Her name is Ms. Linda Thomas.

Granny Gets a New Knee

B.S. (It's not what you think)
It means Before Surgery

Granny's Kitchen

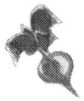 : Jerome?

JEROME …

 : I'm coming, Granny.

 : Pick that bowl up off the floor for me will you, and start shelling the peas in that bag.

 : Then can I shoot some hoops?

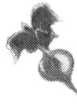 : Did you get your homework done?

 : I did my math and spelling words, and I can do my reading after my shower tonight.

 : You can go play after the peas are shelled and after you water the tomatoes.

 : Deal!

 : Make sure you give those tomatoes a good drink, now. Don't just wave the hose over them. It was a scorcher today.

 : I'll do it like I'm you, Granny.

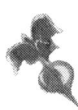 : All right, then.

6 weeks B.S.

First Class With Ms. Linda Or, Soft Shoe Shuffle

 : Just put the milk and eggs in the fridge, Deisha. Leave the taters out, I'll steam them up tonight with my kale salad. I gotta sit down.

 : What did you do in that class?

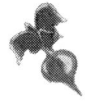 : Listened, mostly. But I learned to do the "Soft Shoe Shuffle" in a chair.

 : Say what?

 : Here, this is what Ms. Linda taught us. Do it with me. Socks on for a wood or tile floor, or barefoot on the carpet.

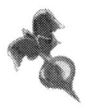 : Put both hands on one thigh and begin to slowly move your other foot forward a little and back, right and left, and in small circles in both directions without losing full contact between the bottom of your foot and the floor.

Keep your knees the same distance apart.

Rest as often as you like, practice on both sides, a little every day. Lighter and lighter. And that's it!

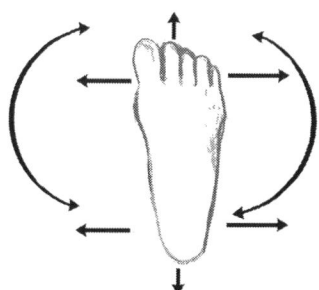

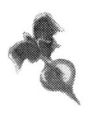 : Ms. Linda says that most pictures used to teach about the human body only show us when we're still. But we're never still, and the best images are the ones we are constantly making and changing in our own heads. She's gonna help me listen to my senses through my skin and muscles and joints and eyes and ears so that my brain pictures are accurate. Then my movement will be more accurate too.

 : < Slam!>

 : Hey Mom. Hey Granny. Can I go play ball at the park with Winston? His older brother and his friends will be there too.

 : Just make sure you take a break and drink plenty of water. Remember last time you got overheated and couldn't go to your school concert? And be home by 6.

 : I will, thanks, bye.

 : And make sure—

 : <Slam!>

 : —you don't let the door slam.

 : Next time.

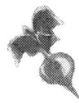 : May be, Deisha. May be.

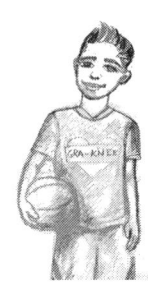 **Jerome's Notes:** You can find the full lesson called *Soft Shoe Shuffle Primer* on Page 86 in Ms. Linda's Class Handouts. I recommend you read her notes starting on Page 78 before you start practicing this or any of the movement lessons. They'll really help you.

Shoes

 : Jerome! Come in here a minute, would you?

Bring all those old shoes out.

 : What are you going to do with them?

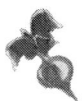 : Give them away. Wait! Not that pair. Hand them up to me.

 : They're dusty.

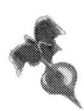 : These were my favorites.

Your Grandpa Gilbert and I used to go dancing every Saturday night.

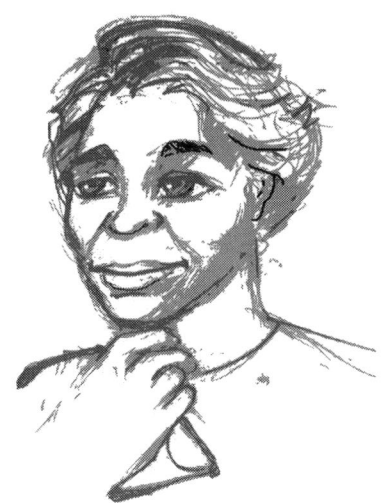

 : You wanna keep em?

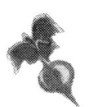 : Put them back in for now, Jerome. The rest of them can go in that big bag.

: But now you've got no shoes, Granny.

 : It's time for new ones.

 : New shoes to go with your new knee?

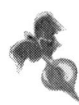 : Something like that, Jerome.

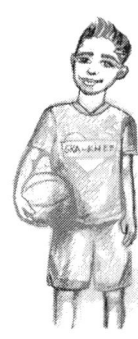 **Jerome's Notes:** Here's what Granny learned to help with her shoe shopping expedition.

What Our Feet Need

A quarter of the bones in the body are in the feet! Take a look.

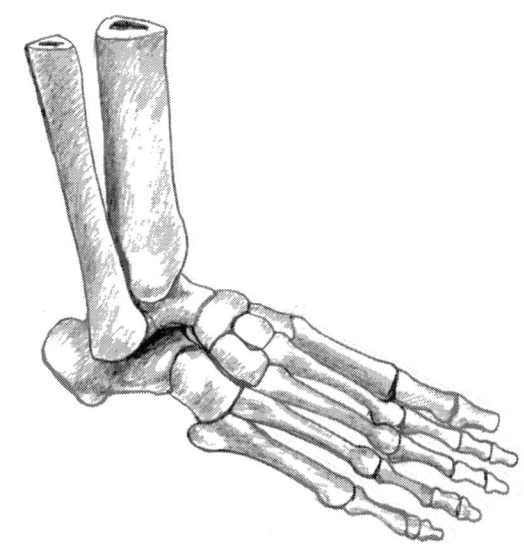

They're meant to move. Not just pointing the toes and bending them back, but rolling side to side. Our shoes need to allow for that.

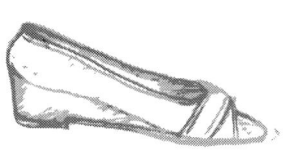
Old walking shoes

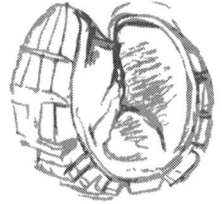
New walking shoes

Shoes that have a stiff piece that goes all the way from the heel to the ball prevent natural movement of the foot, and decrease the stimulation for muscles in the calf, thigh, and back to work effectively against gravity. This can reduce your ability to regain your balance as well.

Try bending the shoe, bringing the toe and heel towards each other across the top. If it is flexible, try it on and walk around in it, keeping the other foot bare to compare. Then put both on and walk around.

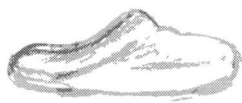 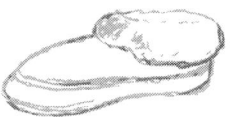

Old slippers   *New slippers*

It's very important that all your shoes have a back or back strap. Otherwise your feet and lower leg muscles overwork trying to stop them from flying off out front or out back.

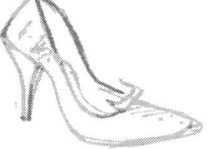 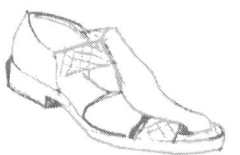

Old fancy shoes   *New fancy shoes*

Constant use of high-heeled shoes reduces the number of ways you use your muscles for walking and the variety of ways the joint surfaces contact each other.

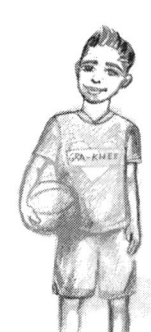

Jerome's Notes: That's the longest shoehorn I've ever seen! This way Granny can put her shoes on without help.

5 weeks B.S.

Second Class
Or, Twist Again

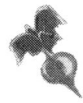 : Ms. Linda says that it's important for me to practice the movement lessons before the surgery, cause afterwards I'll be cleaning out the anesthesia chemicals and managing pain that's different from the pain I've had in my knee all these years.

 : I can help, Granny. Let me do something.

 : I kinda hoped you'd say that, Jerome. Let's see … I have instructions for today's lesson right here, and I need someone to read them out for me.

 : I can do that!

 : I bet you can.

 : These are funny pictures.

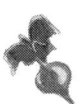 : I think Ms. Linda said they're just to give you an idea of the movement, or a reminder, but they're not the 'right' way.

 : Right. I mean, OK, got it.

 : I've done my scan and I'm on my side, so skip to "A."

 : "Bring your **(R)** knee," what's your **(R)** knee Granny?

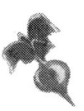 : If you keep reading, you'll see I have a **(L)** knee as well. Is that enough of a clue?

: OK, OK. I got it.

"Bring your right knee away from your left knee and back, keeping your feet together. Now add rolling your head to look right towards the ceiling and back, as you lift your—"

 : Whoa, Whoa, Whoa. I can't keep up.

 : But Granny, you always do everything fast.

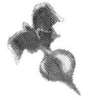 : And look where it's got me! I need to go slow so as to know what I'm doing. Now, start again.

 : That was my first time. I'll get better.

 : That's the idea.

 : "Bring your right knee away from your left knee and back, keeping your feet together.

Pause.

Practice this a few times.

Now add rolling your head to look right…"

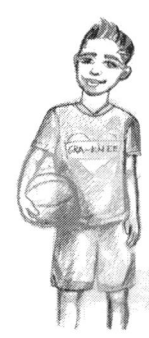 **Jerome's Notes:** When you are ready to try the *Twist Again* lesson, you'll find it in Ms. Linda's Handouts on page 88. You can continue reading her notes if you didn't get through them. They really help!

On page 84 you can read how to do the scan Granny mentions. Doing this before and after each lesson helps you measure your progress.

Twenty Minutes Later ...

 : Uh, Granny, are you asleep?

 : No, Jerome.

 : Did you hear me say to get up and walk around a little?

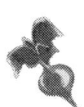 : Yes, Jerome. It's just that I never felt how my spine turns together with my head and pelvis before …

and that my ribs can turn even when my arms are not moving … amazing.

 : People always talk in books and movies about having an "out of body" experience. Sounds like you had an "in body" experience.

 : I like that, Jerome. An "in body" experience. Where else can I be? Really.

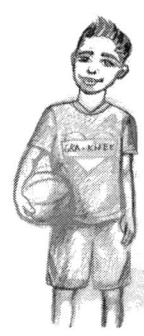

Jerome's Notes: It's time to start building a daily schedule. Start with this, but find what works best for you.

Schedule: Practice *Twist Again* twice a day for 5 – 10 minutes, and practice *Soft Shoe Shuffle* before getting up to walk anywhere.

A Special Note from Granny

Ms. Linda says the only thing all the orthopedic doctors agree on is that walking is the best exercise after surgery. But the way I've been walking all these years was grinding down the bones of my knee, and I didn't even know it! She says that with the new knee, I'll have a new opportunity to improve how I use myself in everything I do, not just walking.

So, I'm learning how to tell where my weight is, so I share the load more evenly and match my muscle effort to my movements. I was working the muscles in my back and legs too hard, more on one side than the other, and had no idea where my hips were.

This is how I found them. Please try this at home.

Stand with your hands on your hips.

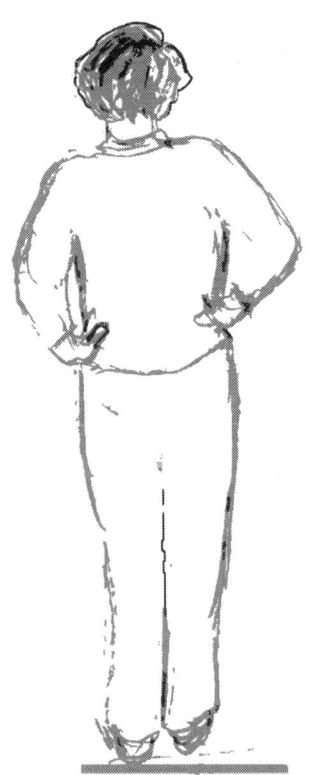

Here's a surprise–your hands are actually on the top of your pelvis! If you keep your thumbs where they are, and swivel your fingers down and out to the side of you, where those dimples are, that's just outside of where your hip joints are.

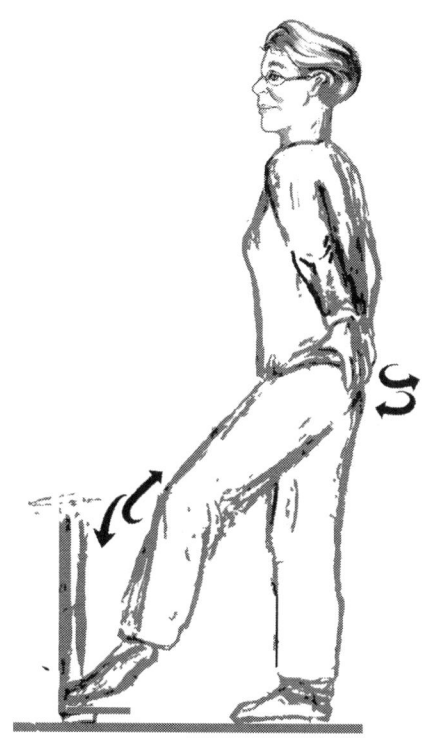

Now put your foot up on a step, and move your knee side to side, while sensing with your fingertips the movement of your hip on that side. Now twist your leg in and out, and sense the movement of your hip.

Walk around a little before you do the same on the other side, and see if your foot contacts the floor differently, or your leg feels lighter, or pushes off more than the other leg.

I still get a kick out of this, and hope you do too. Maybe we'll stop teaching kids to put their hands on their 'hips.'

4 weeks B.S.

Third Class
Or, Helicopter Circles

 : Are you OK, Granny?

 : Uh-huh. Just practicing.

 : Waving your foot around?

 : It may look like that's all that's happening Ernesto, but I can feel movement in my hip, and my back, and all the way up into my chest.

 : I guess we're all connected.

 : And I'm learning how to sense that from the inside. Talking about it is not the same.

 : You've lost me.

 : Try this:

Stand with your feet comfortably apart.

Now put one leg out, as if to take a step,

and keep it out. There's a gap between your foot and the ground.

26 · Granny Gets a New Knee

How can you reach the ground?

Slowly turn around yourself to look at the outside of your standing foot.

Did the leading foot land? The leg can't get any longer, but the pelvis and spine can.

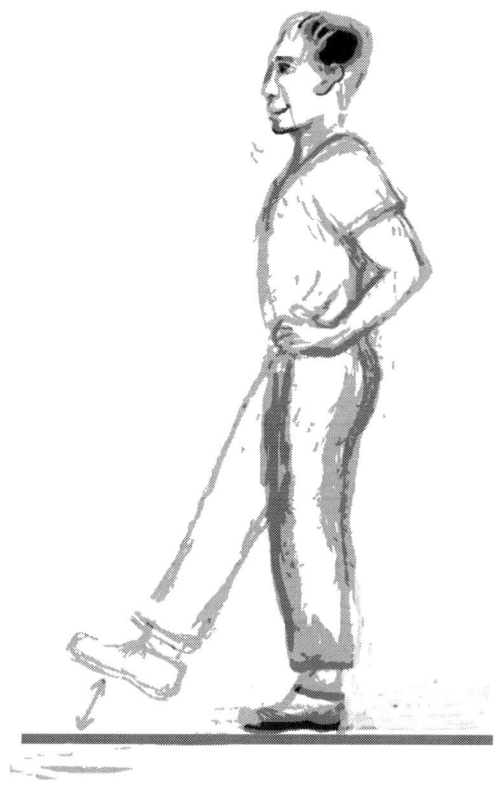

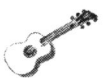 : And this is where the foot waving comes in?

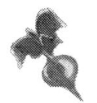 : Sounds silly doesn't it?

Ms. Linda says that we're so used to our talking leading. But we all learned to walk before we could talk, and with no instruction. We were learning how our sensing and moving work together.

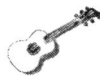 : We're talking ancient history now.

 : You're not such an old dog that you can't learn new tricks, are you?

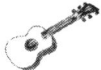 : Well, when you put it like that.

 : You're not getting any younger, why not get smarter?

Give it a try.

 : No time like the present.

 : That's the spirit!

So, lie on your belly …

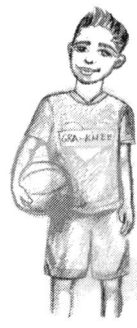

Jerome's Notes: You'll find *Helicopter Circles* on Page 90. Continue scanning your contact before and after each practice. If you need to read Ms. Linda's notes again, go ahead. Remember, you can start with the easier side, even if the instructions start with the Right **(R)** side.

Schedule: Practice this one every morning before you get out of bed and when you first get into bed at night, and continue with *Twist Again*, and *Soft Shoe Shuffle* before walking.

Granny's First Acupuncture Visit — Ever!

B.A.
Before Acupuncture

(Were you looking at the picture first? Yikes!)

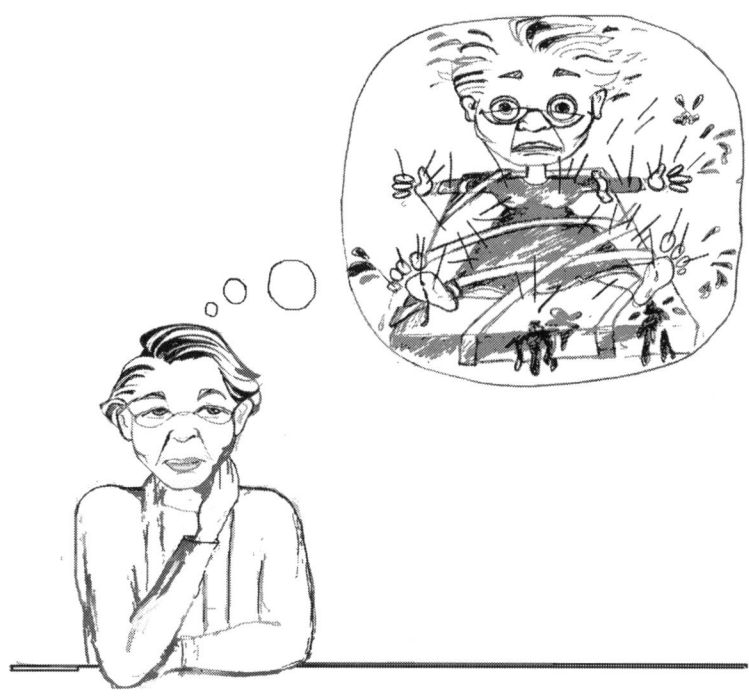

 : Would you like me to come in with you?

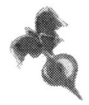 : I'm still not sure I'm going in.

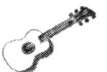 : We can just sit here. You let me know when you're ready, or if you want to go home.

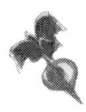 : But I said I'd try it, we all did, and Mary Jane did it on Monday … and said it didn't really hurt at all … and the needles were sterilized … and she felt stuff moving inside her in a good way … and then she fell asleep for two hours.

 : <Sigh>

 : Oh come on. Let's do this.

A.A.

After Acupuncture

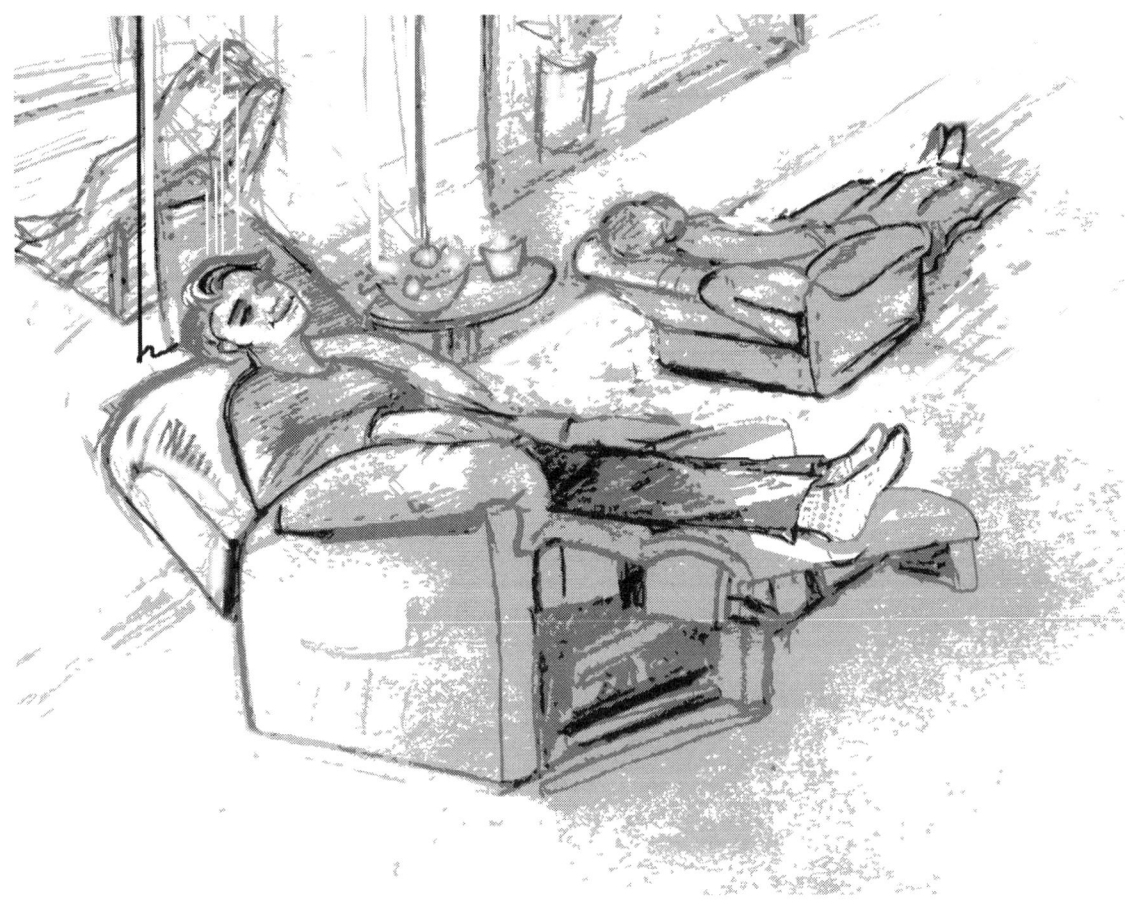

3 weeks B.S.

Fourth Class
Or, Climbing the Walls

 : Tell me. Why am I here again? I'm the only kid.

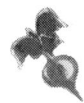 : I thought you'd like to see what goes on, first hand. 'Sides, everyone has a surgery buddy, and I'd like you to be mine.

 : Awh. You sure know how to get me, Granny. You musta known me a long time, huh.

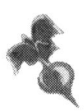 : All your life, Jerome. All your life.

Here's Ms. Linda.

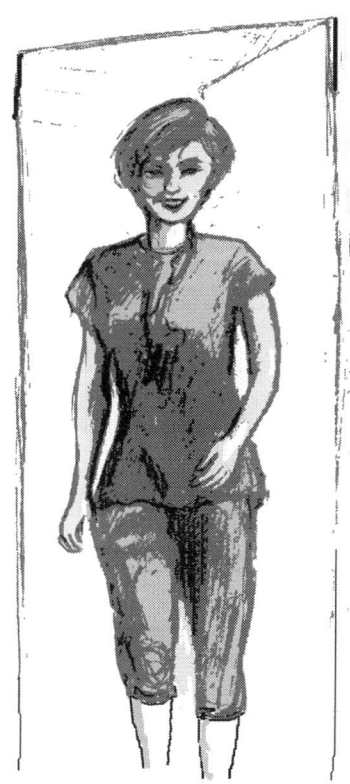

Granny Gets a New Knee · 31

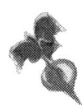 : Ms. Linda, this here's my grandson, Jerome.

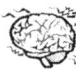 : Lovely to meet you Jerome. I hear you've been helping your Granny with her lessons and a whole lot more.

 : Um, yeah, I guess.

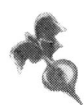 : He sure has.

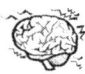 : Would you like to join us for today's lesson? I think you might enjoy this one.

 : Welcome everyone. I'm ready to begin.
Please, find a place in front of the wall, making space for each other, about arm distance apart from your neighbors …

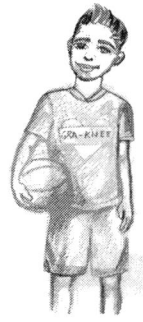

Jerome's Notes: You'll find *Climbing the Walls* on page 92.

Schedule: Practice this every day or every other day for two to three minutes, depending on your pain level while standing. Continue with the other lessons each day, so that you become comfortable with focusing on your moving for longer periods of time.

Later ...

 : This salad is *delicioso*, Dad.

 : *Gracias*, Jerome. Who's going first with news?

 : I had school.

 : Yes, and ... ?

 : Just regular.

 : Didn't you—

 : Oh, we started drawing our characters for our Gold Rush comics and I drew this one old guy and a younger guy ...

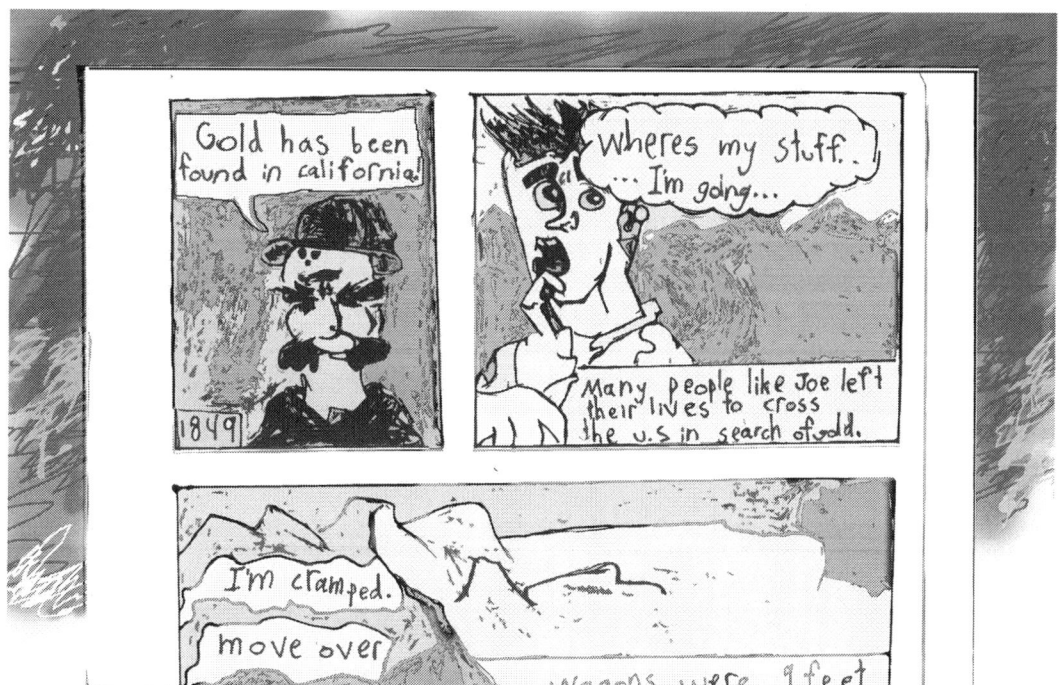

 : They're quite the characters, *m'ijo*.

: I like this one's mustache.

 : …And then I went to class with Granny and did the lesson with Ms. Linda, and you know, after I did that lesson, I think I got taller! I mean I feel taller and lighter and can one of you come outside and shoot some baskets with me after dinner? Please?

 : You know, I've been cooped up all day re-writing this chapter. I'll shoot a few with you.

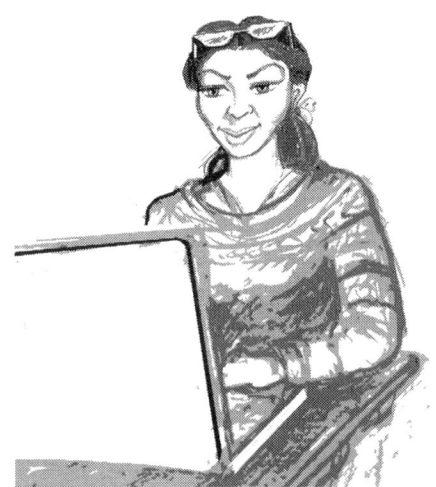

 : Great. Dad?

 : Maybe after I clean up the kitchen.

 : OK. But if I hear the guitar, I'm coming to get you.

 : Fair enough.

 : Before we start, do you think you could show me what you did in class? I could do with a little 'lighter.'

 : Sure. I bet it'll help with your headaches, too.

 : May be, Jerome. May be.

Preparations

 : I'm going up to the store, Mom. Do you need me to pick up your pain pills?

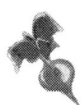 : I don't think so. Could you check and see how many I have left? I think they're up in my bathroom.

 : I'll look, but they're usually down there with you.

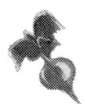 : Not lately.

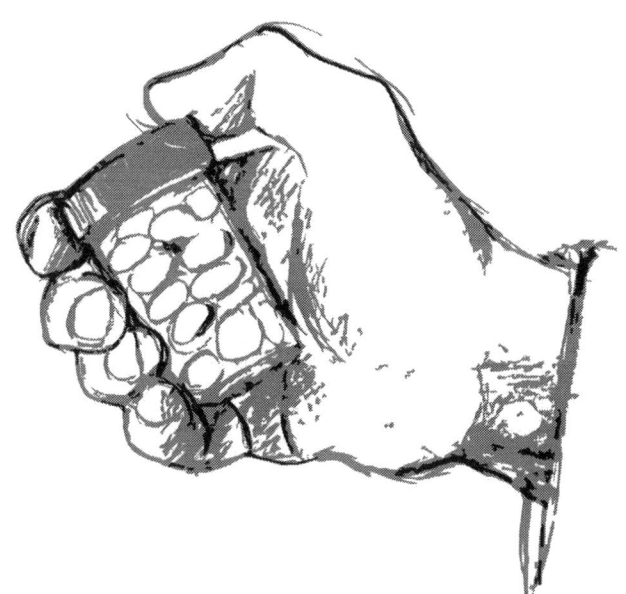

 : It's almost full.

 : Don't sound so surprised. Since I've been practicing my lessons I haven't needed to take as many as I used to.

 : Sounds like great motivation to keep practicing.

 : It is. Anyway, I have to stop taking them completely about 4 days before the surgery. They're anti-inflammatory pills.

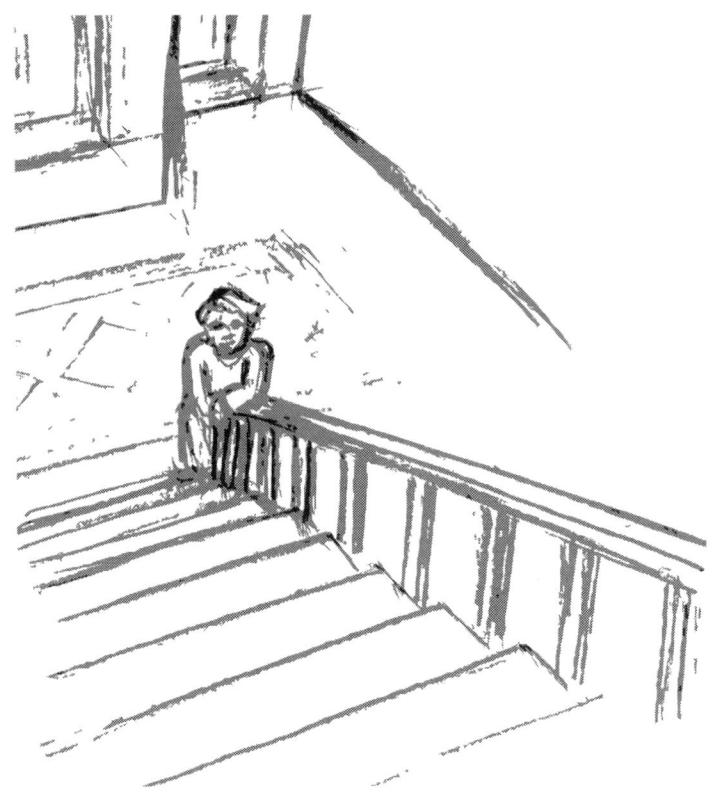

 : Hey Mom, are you going to be able to do these stairs when you come home?

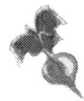 : Oh no, honey. I'll be sleeping down here for a while. Delora will sleep up there the week she's here.

 : You seem to have it all covered.

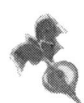 : I've had a lot of help, and I'll need a lot too.

 : We're here for you, Ma.

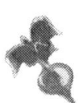 : I know, Deisha. I know.

2 weeks B.S.

Fifth Class
Or, First Movements

 : Granny, how do they get the new knee in?

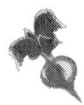 : They make an incision, or cut, down the front and replace the worn out surfaces of the femur and tibia. See here:

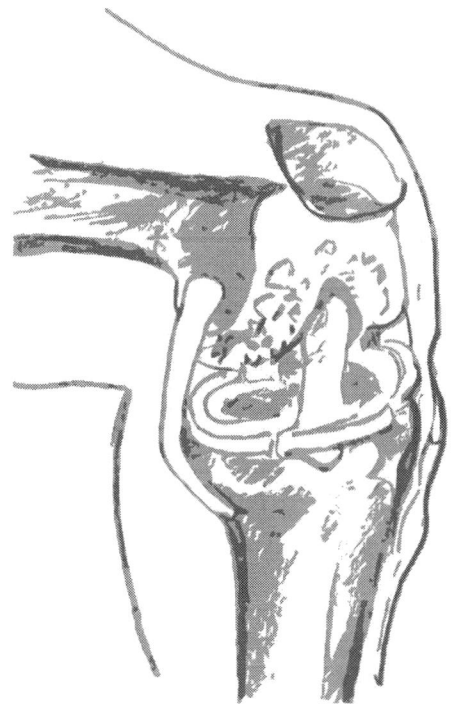

Before

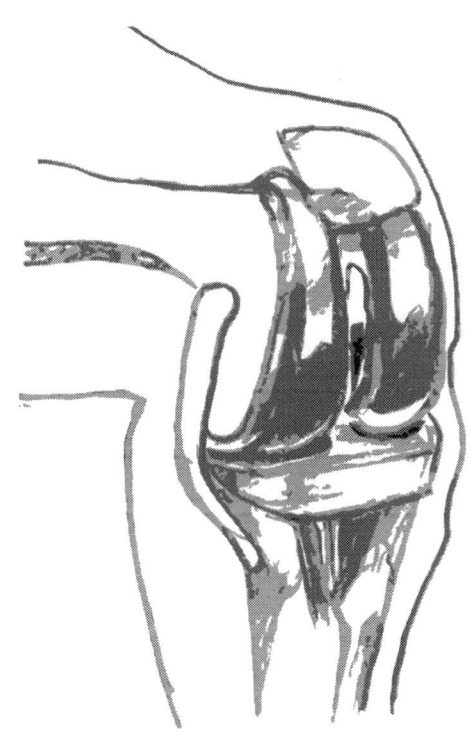

After

 : What do they replace them with?

 : Metal parts and a plastic cushion.

 : How do they stay there?

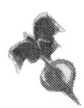 : In my case, with special fast-curing medical cement so I can get up and put some weight on this leg straight away.

 : Straight away?!! But don't you need to rest?

 : Yes. But I need to start walking to move my knee and to help with the circulation, because my chances of making a **DVT** are greater if—

 : You're gonna make a movie?

 : Not a **DVD**. A **DVT**. A **D**eep **V**ein **T**hrombosis.

 : A what?

 : That's when the blood in the leg slows down and bits of tissue from the surgery can clump together to form a clot, and if it gets big enough, it can block the whole vein.

 : That doesn't sound good.

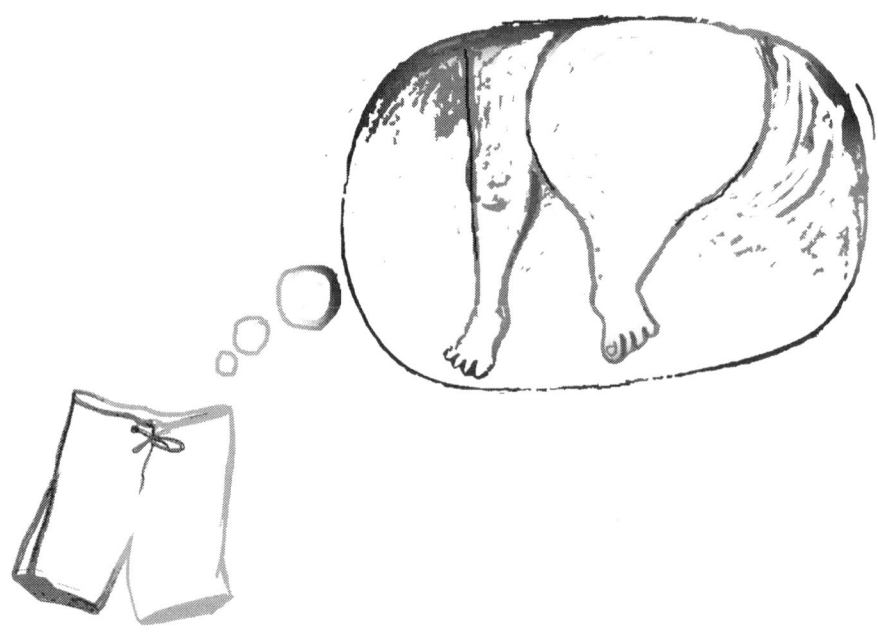

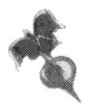 : There's more. If it gets loose and travels up through the heart and gets stuck in the smaller vessels of the lungs, it's called a Pulmonary Embolism, and then the blood backs up into the heart and—

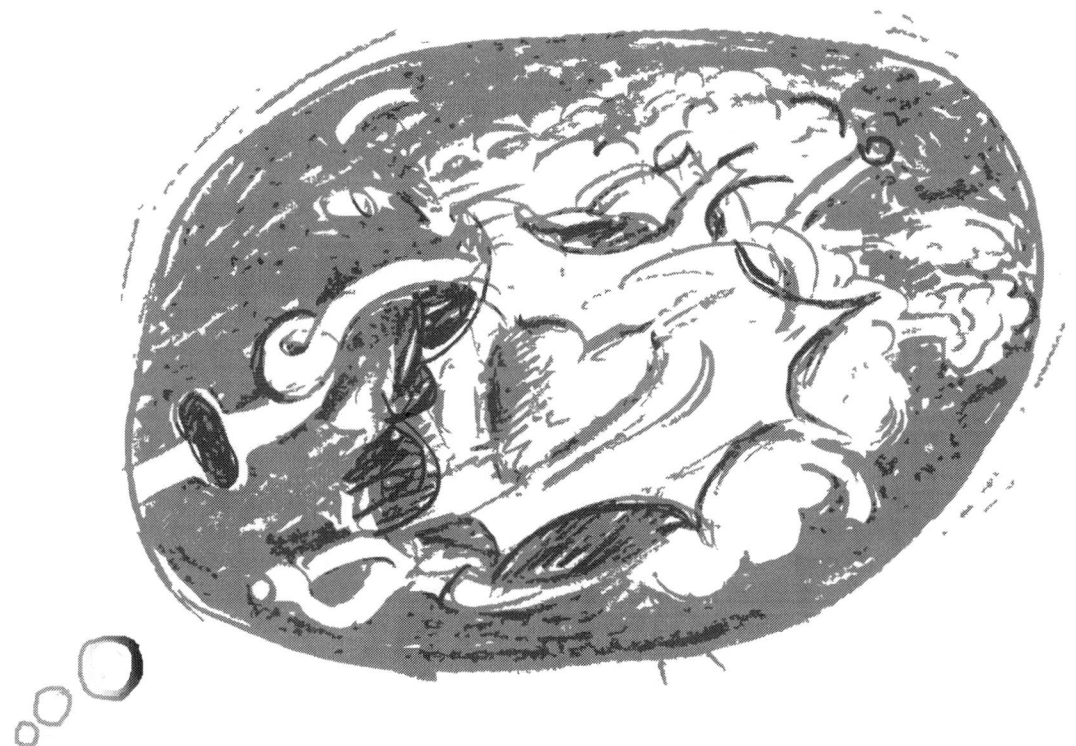

 : That REALLY doesn't sound good.

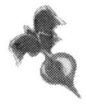 : Not at all. So that's why these movements from today's class are so important.

 : Well, what are we waiting for?

 : Well, your next question.

 : OK. OK. I'm done.

Granny?

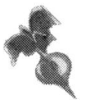 : Yes, Jerome?

: I think you're really brave.

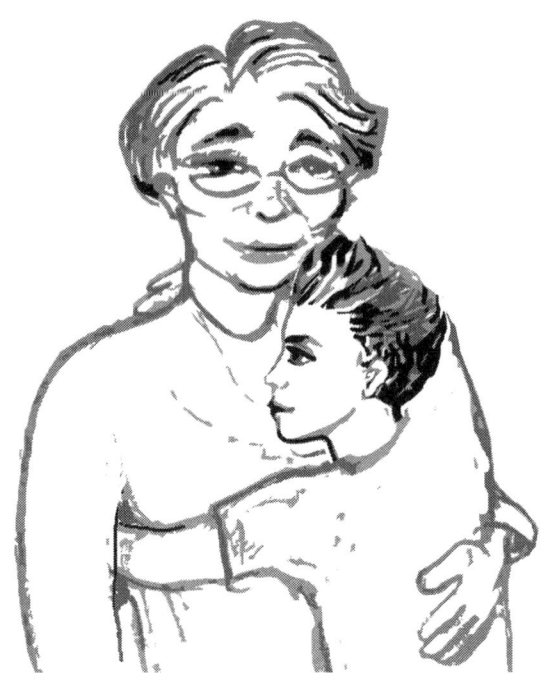

 : Now, let's get practicing. Please "lie on your back …"

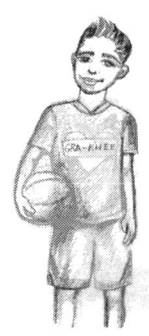 **Jerome's Notes:** You'll find *First Movements* on page 94. Practice these movements as if you have had the surgery, and you need to move very slowly and carefully.

Schedule: Take a look at the suggested daily schedules for after the surgery on page 102, and begin to practice them. Be familiar with both the hospital and at home schedules.

Later ...

 : Have you flossed, Jerome?

 : Brushed?

 : Yup, Yup.

 : Are you reading?

 : Mmmmmmmmmmmm.

 : Put it down. Now, *m'ijo*.

 : Just a minute—

 : Now.

 : <Snatch>

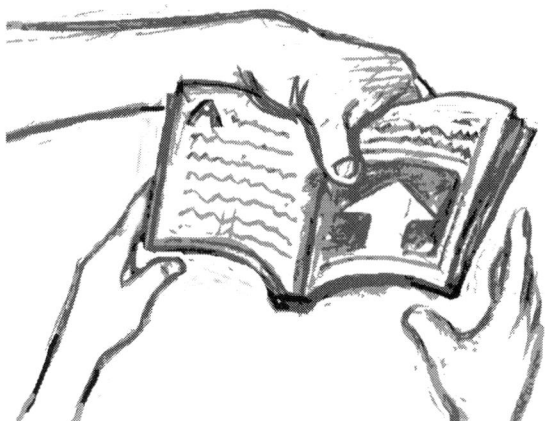

 : Hands.

With our hands we form a family circle of safety.

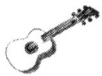 : A family circle of safety.

: Ohhhhhhh Kay.

  : Good night. Sleep tight. I love you.

 : <Click>

 : Thank you, Jerome.

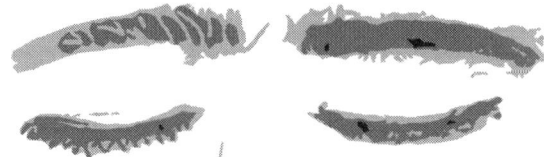

 : You're welcome.

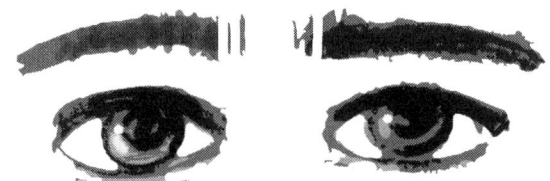

 : What for?

 : Taking such good care of your Granny.

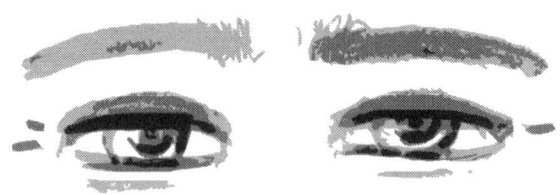

 : *De nada*, Mami.

10 days B.S.

TLAs

 : Ms. Linda? Could you explain to Jerome about the **INR**? He's really worried about the **DVT**.

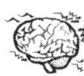 : All those **TLA**s are enough to confuse and worry anyone.

 : **TLA**s?

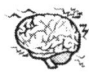 : **T**hree **L**etter **A**cronyms.

Like **TKA** for **T**otal **K**nee **A**rthroplasty or **TKR** for **T**otal **K**nee **R**eplacement. It's like short hand.

So, **INR** stands for **I**nternational **N**ormalized **R**atio and it's a measure of how quickly or slowly your blood clots.

 : We don't want Granny's blood to clot too quickly—

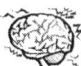 : Or too slowly, otherwise any cut or bump will continue to bleed.

 : So it's gotta be juuuuuuuuust right.

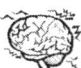 : Within a narrow range, yes. That's why before and for a couple of weeks after surgery, Granny needs to stop eating foods high in Vitamin **K**, because they help with clotting.

 : What kind of foods?

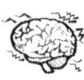 : The **K**ings of **K** are kale, collards, and spinach. Also turnip, beet, and mustard greens, broccoli, and brussels sprouts. And green tea too.

 : Uh, oh. Granny loves her kale and collards.

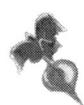 : You said I can eat coleslaw and salads with chickpeas and squash and carrots and cauliflower, right Ms. Linda?

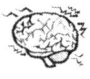 : Absolutely. You just need to use measured amounts consistently so we can keep you in the 'just right' range with your medication. That'll be measured every couple of days after surgery. Make sense, Jerome?

 : Uh-huh.

But how long do we have to look out for the **DVT**?

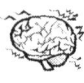 : We'll keep a close eye after surgery, then you need to be watchful once your Granny comes home, especially ten days or so after surgery. About three months total.

 : What will we be looking for?

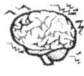 : Sudden swelling in either leg, muscle tenderness that's new, change in skin color, or increase in warmth. If you're not sure, always call to get help.

 : Phew, this is a big project.

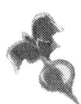 : Too much for you, Jerome?

: No way, Granny. You're worth it. I know how much you want to get out in the garden.

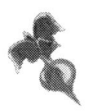 : Ain't that the truth, Jerome. Ain't that the truth.

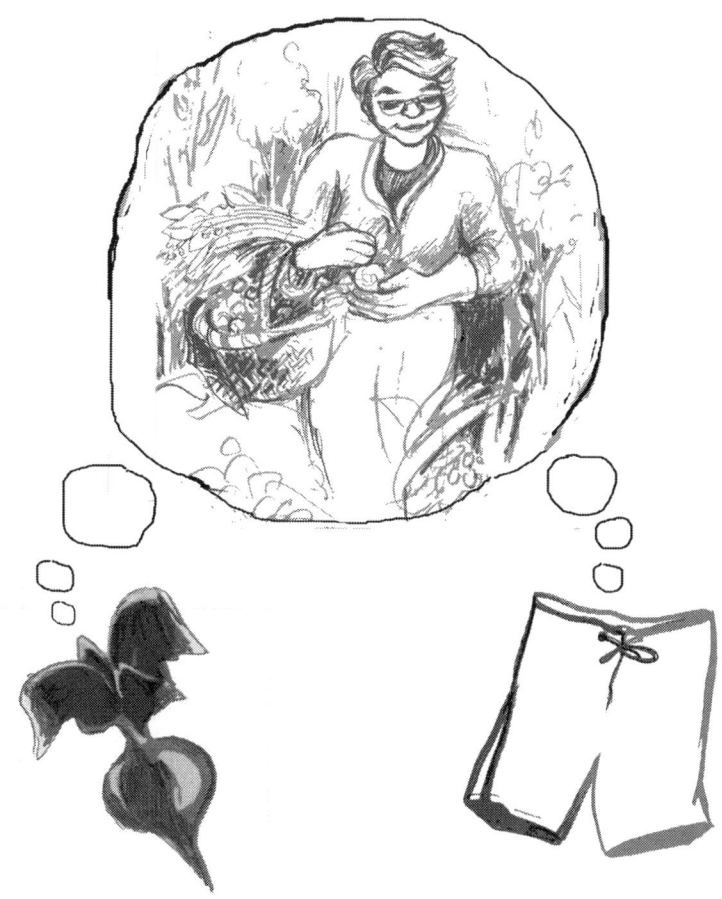

1 week B.S.

Sixth Class
Or, The Floor is My Friend

 : What are you doing, Granny?

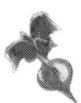 : What does it look like?

 : Like when Mom and Dad get silly and pretend they're playing that game from when they were young.

 : Twister?

 : Yeah, that's the one. But why are you doing it?

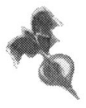 : I'm actually practicing some movements that will gradually help me get down to the floor and back up again. That's what we did in class yesterday.

 : But you don't need to get down, Granny. I can take care of anything on the floor.

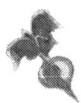 : I appreciate that Jerome, but—

 : But Ms. Linda says?

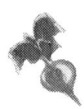 : Yes, Jerome, that's very funny. BUT, it's not just about picking things up off the floor. When we were in the lesson yesterday with our behinds up in the air, someone started to giggle, and pretty soon we were all laughing, and I'm not sure why exactly, but it felt really good. I haven't laughed like that in years.

: So what shall we call this one? Bellyache? Side-splitter?

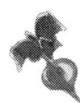 : I think maybe 'Second Childhood.'

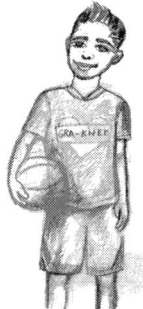

Jerome's Notes: You'll find *The Floor is My Friend* on page 96.

Schedule: Practice progressing slowly through this lesson every other day. It doesn't even matter if you don't get to the floor before or after the surgery. Practice doing what you can, comfortably. You can pick it up again after the surgery, when you are ready; it'll be different for each person. Continue to practice the other lessons too, following the suggested schedule on page 104 or making up your own.

4 days B.S.

Lists and Logistics

 : Cooool! Where'd you get all the stuff, Granny?

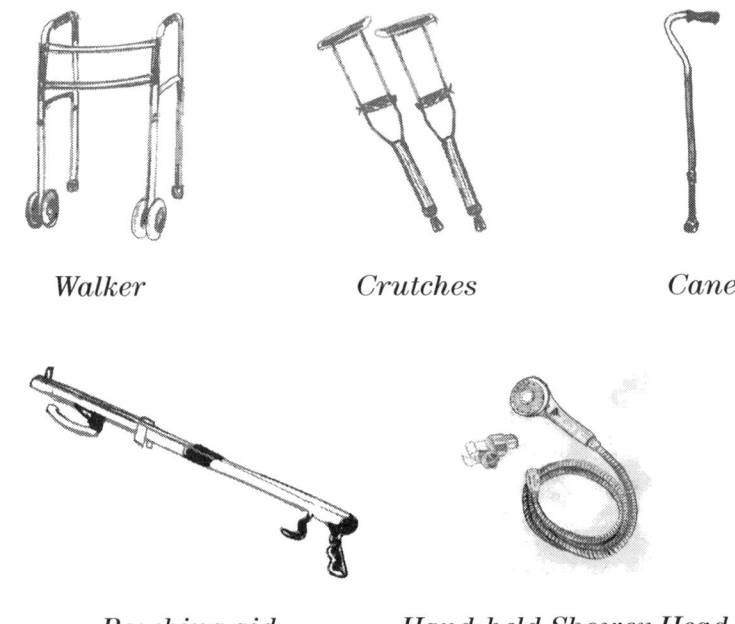

 : It just got delivered, and the hospital bed will arrive just before I come home.

If you're gonna play with those crutches, you need to adjust them so your elbows are straight and there's a space under your armpit. That's right. Now change the length from the bottom—

 : My arms are too skinny—

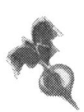 : Your arms are just fine, Jerome.

You gotta hug the top against your ribs; don't lean on it or you could damage your nerve. Think of carrying your weight through your bones.

---

48 · Granny Gets a New Knee

Would you put this commode over the toilet and this plastic stool in the shower while your arms are still functioning?

 : *No problema.*

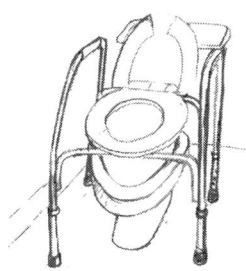   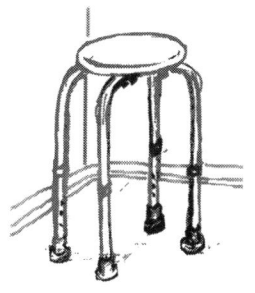

Commode over the toilet   *Adjustable height shower stool*

 : Now, we have some things to take care of. This is my list:

> *Garden–watering, weeding*
>
> *Grocery shopping*
>
> *Cooking*
>
> *Laundry*
>
> *Dusting/vacuuming*
>
> *Trash, recycling, emptying compost bins*
>
> *All bins out Wednesdays*
>
> *Paying bills*
>
> *Visiting with Mrs. Lawton*

 : That's an awfully long list, Granny. I guess grown-ups have a lot of stuff to do.

 : Too much, and I need to delegate most of this so I can concentrate on my movement lessons after the surgery.

 : You can put me down for the garden and I'll get Dad to do the trash, recycling, and compost with me. Even though it stinks.

Granny Gets a New Knee

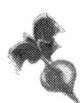 : Thanks, Jerome. You're a *mensch*.

 : A what?

 : A kind person, a good person.

 : I'm a *mensch*.

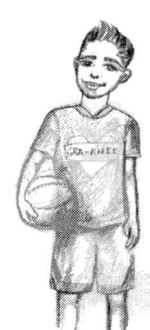

Jerome's Notes: You'll find the list of equipment in Ms. Linda's notes on page 112.

Look for these symbols above the titles in the chapters after surgery to see which walking aids Granny is using:

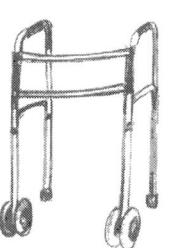 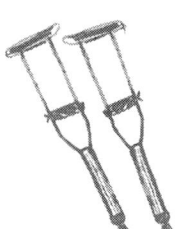 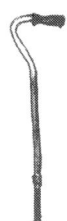

Granny Goes in for Surgery

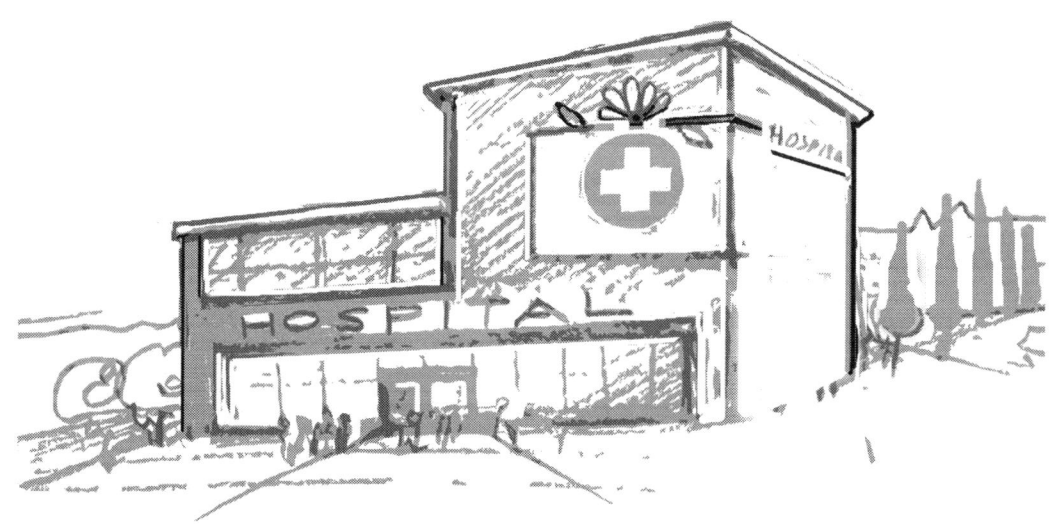

 : You've got your toothbrush and tooth goop here with your floss sticks, pants with baggy legs, oh, and don't forget to start doing your first movements as soon as you wake up afterwards, even if it's just imagining them or making tiny movements, or moving on the other side first, and—

 : Deisha!

I'm gonna be OK. They've done thousands of these, it's only me that's a novice, and I'm ready. We've been preparing for weeks.

 : You're right. I know.

It's just …

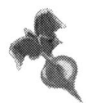 : Family circle?

 : Sure.

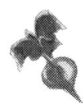 : With our hands we form a family circle of safety.

 : A family circle of safety.

 : Ohhhhhhh-Kay.

 : I love you, Mom.

 : I love you, D.

A.S.
After Surgery

Sanchez Kitchen

 : That's the formula for finding the area, not the perimeter. You know this stuff, Jerome. What's going on?

 : Nothing.
It's just that I've got a lot of homework this week.

 : Are you thinking about Granny?

 : It's not that.
Well, yes, I guess I am a little distracted.

 : I told you, Jerome. She came through the surgery fine; she started moving in Recovery before anyone even reminded her.

 : That sounds like Granny.
Is she in a lot of pain?

 : They're doing a good job managing that. They even have a special machine that pumps icy water around her knee and they helped her get up and walk to the bathroom today.

 : Just like we practiced.

 : That's right, and as soon as she can walk up and down the hallway and go up and down a few steps, she'll be coming home, probably tomorrow or the next day.

 : And that's when Delora and I will be up.

: You two have made Granny's downstairs area so cozy. She'll have everything she needs at her fingertips.

 : At her reacher tips, you mean.

 : Yes. At her reacher tips.

Jerome's Notes:

I… ☐ hope

☐ pray

☐ cross my fingers

☐ trust

☐ am sure   …the new knee will work.

Day 2

Practice, Practice, Practice

 : Hey Jerome.

 : Hey Delora. Finished your paper?

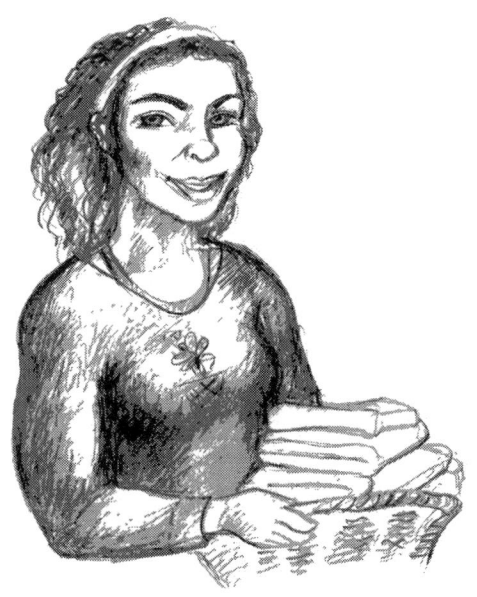

 : Just about. Thought I'd take a break and maybe get you to go over those lessons with me.

 : Sure, and then shoot some hoops? Mom? I can do my reading before bed.

 : You've got about forty minutes before your dad gets home and we eat dinner.

 : Yes!

 : I'll just put this load of towels in the washer.

: One just finished. Would you hang them out on the line for me?

 : Sure thing, Auntie D.

 : I'm gonna put my new shorts on.

 : OK.

He's so grown up, Auntie D. So 'in charge.'

 : Isn't he? This whole knee thing has given them both so much confidence.

 : You must be so pleased for him.

 : I am, Delora. I am.

Day 4

Revolving Door

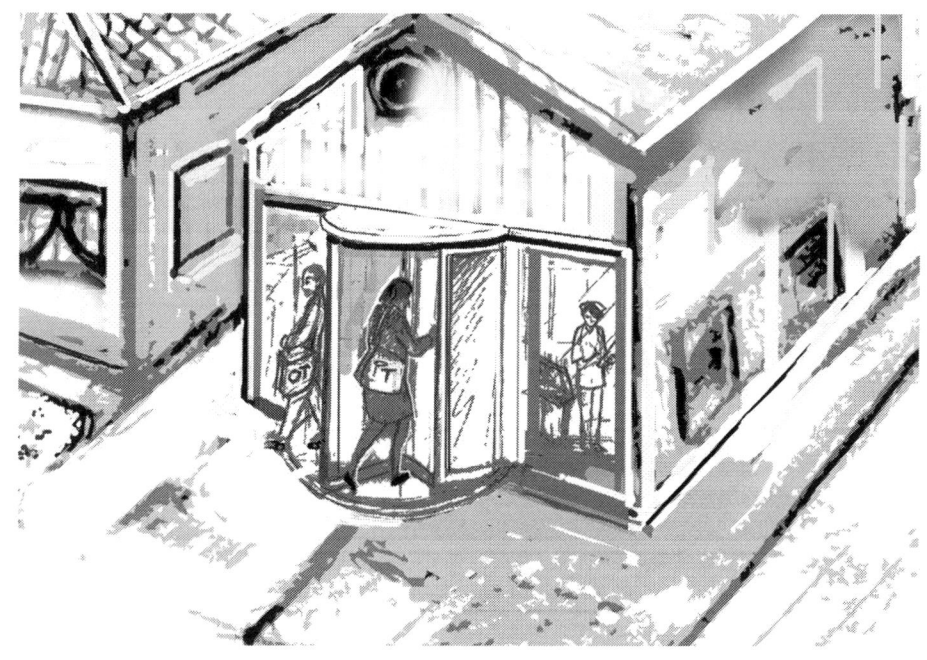

 : Hello. Yes, please come in … I will … thank you. Tomorrow? What time? Yes, I know how to use the ice—all the way around the knee for 15 to 20 minutes at least three to four times a day, or as tolerated. And yes, I'll take out all the small area rugs so that she won't get stuck and trip… Yes, I'll make sure she continues with the lessons every day…

Phew.

I didn't realize there'd be so much coming and going.

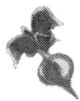 : It won't last long. Everyone says I'm doing great. I just feel so tired.

 : Let's get you settled for a nap.

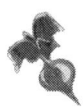 : I need to walk around a bit first. I've been sitting too long and my knee's a little stiff.

: Your workout rivals what we do at school, Granny. I'm impressed.

 : Wait till you see my Soft Shoe Shuffle.

 : Your what?

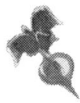 : I need to do some before I walk–it goes like this …

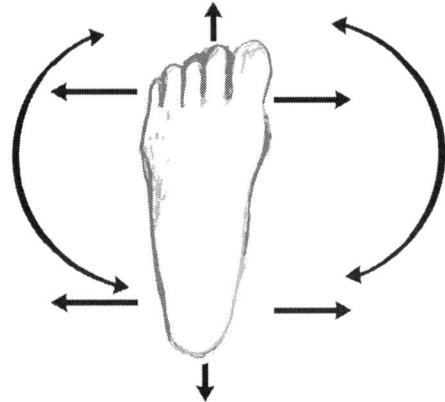

Day 5

Practice Buddies

 : Why's this one called 'Climbing the Walls,' Granny?

 : 'Cause Ms. Linda said we'd be feeling this way about now, so why not match the feeling to the words and the words to the action.

 : Sorta Shakespearean.

 : Make sure you move your eyes slowly and with the turning of your spine. Think of your eyes as the top of your spine.

 : I don't get it.

 : Be patient, this is different. Be like an explorer in a new world rather than a commuter taking the same trip over and over.

 : I can't go up the wall as far with this hand, but if I try harder—

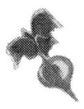 : If you can't go as far, something in you is stopping the movement and if you try harder, it's just you against you, and you'll lose. Go as far as you can, easily.

Pause there, breathe.

Go back and forth, a tiny movement, a few times.

When you rock forward on your foot, do your ribs and chin move up?

Does your chest move closer to the wall?
Can you feel a line from your foot through to your opposite hand?

: How do you know all this?

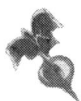 : Jerome and I have been practicing, and each time, I learn something new, something I didn't know before.

 : Like what?

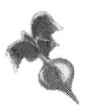 : Like pushing harder.

I used to do that all the time.

Now I ask, 'which part of me is resisting or not participating?' Like in a team, you're gonna have more fun if everyone is playing well together.

 : That, I do know.

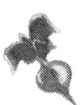 : Let's walk a bit. We'll come back to this tomorrow.

Day 6
Breathing Up and Down

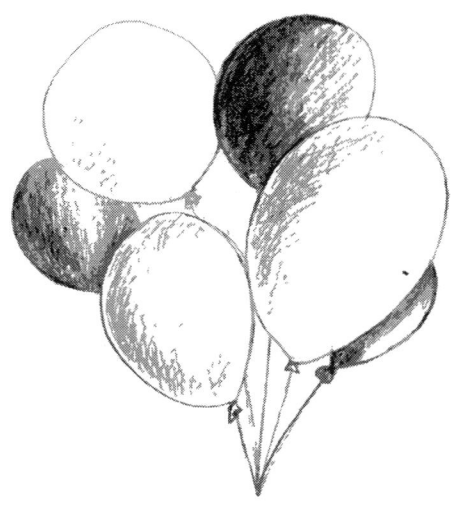

 : Is this a party I didn't know about?

 : As if. Grab a balloon and join us.

 : First, he needs to do a couple sit-to-stand-to-sits. Slowly.

 : Not the 'comfy' chair, Uncle Neto. Try the wooden one, and sit on the front edge.

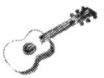 : Not you too! Isn't it enough having Jerome and your Granny channeling Ms. Linda?

 : My turn!

Notice whether your knees move forward as you begin to stand. Where are your eyes looking? Do you hold your breath?

 : I'm supposed to notice all that AND move?

 : You've been able to do both together since you were a baby, Neto. You're just out of practice, like most adults.

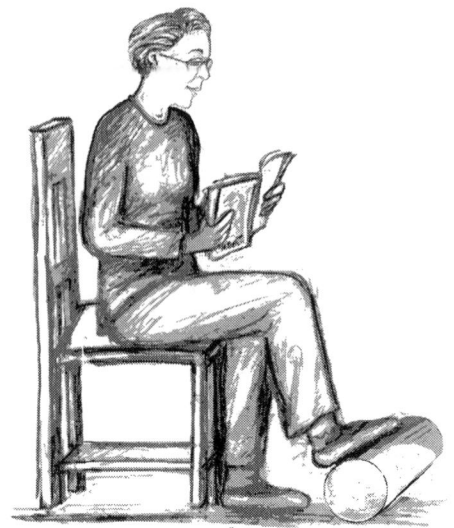

 : Now everyone, without taking a deep breath, blow all your air out into the balloon and release it.

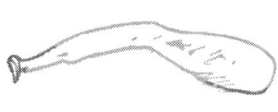 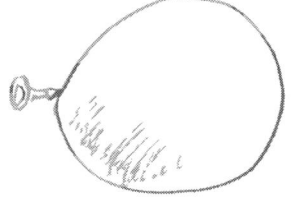

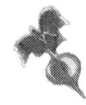 : Do it again, and as you blow into the balloon, slowly begin to move towards sitting, looking down the wall in front of you, towards the floor. When all your air is pushed out, let fresh air rush back in, bringing you up to standing, your eyes coming up the wall from the floor. Like a spring uncoiling.

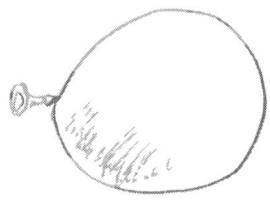 THEN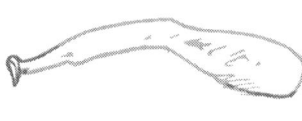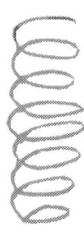

 : This time, breathe in as you move towards sitting, then push the air into the balloon as you stand up slowly. Out of your ribs in all directions, your belly and your low back.

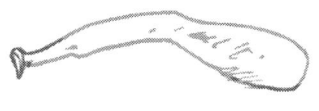 THEN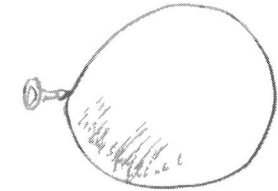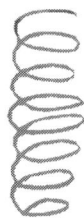

 : Now do it the first way again. Breathing out as you move down, in as you spring up.

 : Put the balloon down, and slowly sit and stand several times. Is this easier? Lighter? Faster? Do you breathe in or out on the way up? On the way down? Can you make it easy to do either? And walk around a little.

Or run and jump, as Jerome likes to do.

 : <Slam!>

 : I had a hard time blowing up my balloon as I was moving up to standing.

 : Me too! But it was easier on the way down, and at warm-ups they always have us focus on breathing in, but pushing all the air out made breathing in feel like no work at all.

 : <Slam!>

 : I touched the bottom of the net for the first time! I'm gonna do it again!

: <Slam!>

 : Jerome!

 : Sorry!

 : How often do you do this, Mom? Doesn't it hurt your knee?

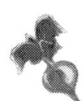 : I don't bend down very far, or do it over and over, but now I connect my breathing whenever I sit down or get up. It helps. Like the balloon is inside me and floats me up.

 : You must be Ms. Linda's poster child.

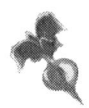 : You'd be surprised. I bet there are families all over saying the same thing.

 : And all just as grateful as we are.

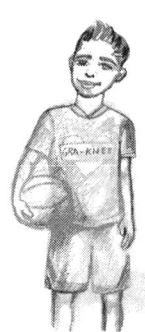

Jerome's Notes: We used balloons, but you can practice this without them.

Did you see that Granny is using a roller to keep moving while she's sitting? She also straightens her knee with her heel on the roller and lengthens her leg out and back. Both sides, like all the lessons. You can do that too.

Day 7 — Delora's 'Back to School' Dinner

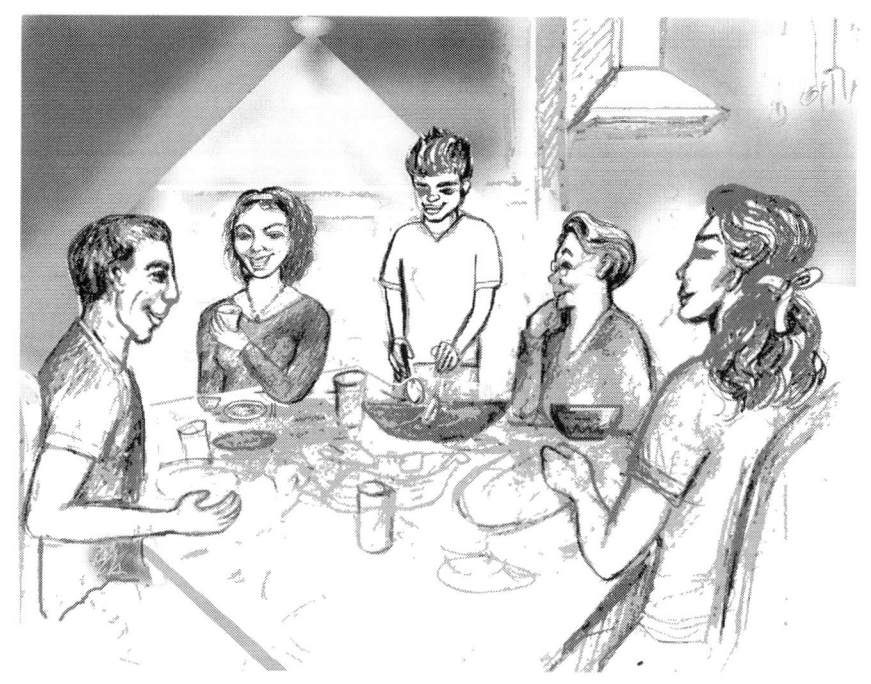

 : Pass the tortillas please, Delora.

 : How many is that now?

 : I'm a growing boy.

 : That'll work better if you add the beans, rice, and cheese.

 : *No problema. Y salsa por favor, Mami.*

 : You'll be doing Granny a favor if you eat all the leftovers. With all the food people have been bringing, there's no space left in her fridge.

 : People have been so kind. Others in my class are not so blessed.

: What do they do?

 : Prepare their own meals before the surgery and freeze them. Some who need extra time to recover go to a rehabilitation facility.

 : Maybe I could hire myself out as a surgery buddy and help with the lessons and food and stuff.

 : You might want to expand your repertoire first.

 : Scrambled eggs, tacos, PB and J. What more do you need?

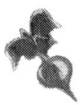 : Mr. Hotshot for hire, I need my ice pack from the freezer, thank you. It's been a long day.

 : On it!

 : We've got clean up, Granny.

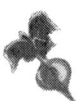 : Truly blessed.

Day 8

Snap

 : Who put these towels in here? They're all wrong; this shouldn't be here, Jerome! Jerome! How can I get what I need when it's down there? Jerome! Oh, there you are. Didn't I tell you to fold these three ways? They don't fit in properly—

 : But Granny, I didn't—

 : I said, THEY DON'T ALL FIT IF YOU DON'T FOLD THEM IN THREE.

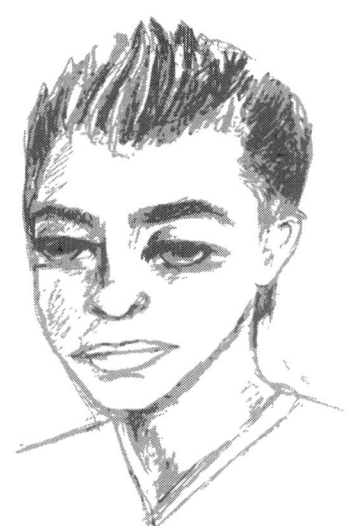

 : \<Nothing but the sounds of the nearby freeway\>

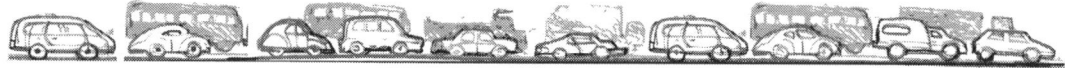

 : \<Sniff, Sniff … Sniff\>

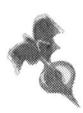 : Jerome. I'm sorry. I need to rest.

Granny Gets a New Knee

: That's OK, Granny.

 : <Deep breath … and the sounds of the nearby freeway>

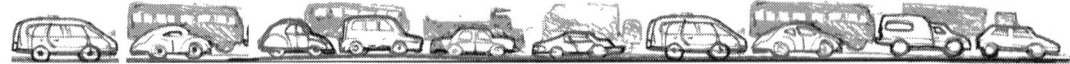

 : Do you think visiting with everyone yesterday was too much? You were sitting still for an awfully long time.

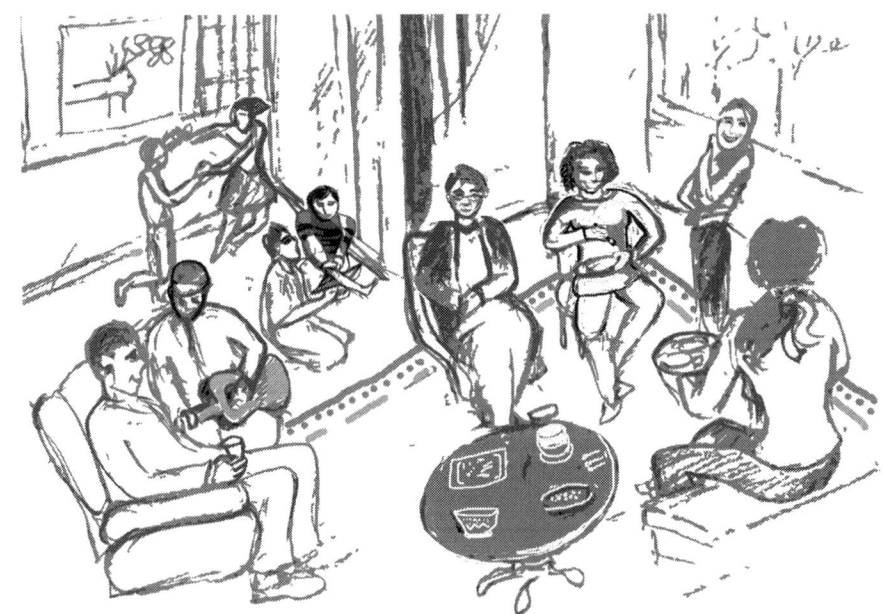

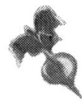 : Maybe, Jerome. But right now I need to put my feet up. Will you please get me the frozen peas from the freezer and my towel?

 : Sure, Granny.

Day 10
All the Way Up

 : Mom? Where are you? MOM?

 : I'm up here, Deisha. I'm upstairs.

 : You went up by yourself?

 : Yes I did.

 : But what if—

 : I went slowly and carefully, just like I've been practicing all along, and now that you're here, we can go back down together.

 : Hey Granny, does this mean we're moving you back upstairs?

 : Not yet, Jerome. Going up and down once is not the same as doing it several times a day. But soon. I sure am looking forward to sleeping in my own bed again.

 : I bet Ms. Linda will be surprised to see you doing so well.

 : I don't know about that, but I think she'll be happy for me.

 : Oh, I nearly forgot. I came over to ask you some important questions. Ready?

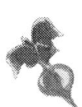 : Ask away.

Granny Gets a New Knee

: Any sudden swelling?

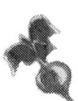 : No.

 : Any new pain or increased warmth?

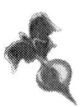 : No, and no again.

 : Any change in skin color?

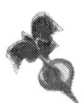 : No. No sign of the dreaded DVT monster, but thanks for being on the lookout.

 : Just doing my job, Granny. Just doing my job.

Day 21 and

First Outing

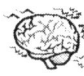 : Ms. Mattie!

Congratulations! I see you've been practicing your lessons and listening to yourself.

 : I have, Ms. Linda.

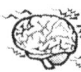 : And using one crutch on the opposite side?

 : I still don't understand why, but it feels better.

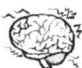 : That's all that matters. Any questions?

 : Yes. When can I start driving again?

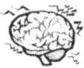 : Ah.

 : You've heard that one before.

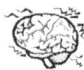 : Once or twice.
   Automatic?

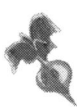 : That's right.

 : Let's get you on our simulator.

Did you get into the passenger seat OK today?

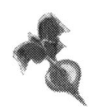 : Just fine.

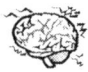 : Great. So, try the driver's seat.

Same as the passenger side, sit, then bring your inside leg in.

Then your outside leg in. You can push down on the steering wheel.

OK. Now practice moving your foot from accelerator to brake and back. Slowly at first, then build up the speed.

Now add in turning the steering wheel … use the indicators … looking out the front … turning to look over one shoulder … then the other.

Lovely. Next time we'll turn on the screen so you can respond to real traffic situations.

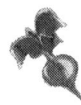 : You forget how complicated it all is—

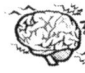 : And you've re-organized so much of your movement—

 : And I notice more now—

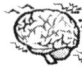 : And if we keep finishing each other's sentences—

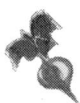 : I'll have to get a job here!

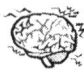 : Wouldn't that be a hoot!

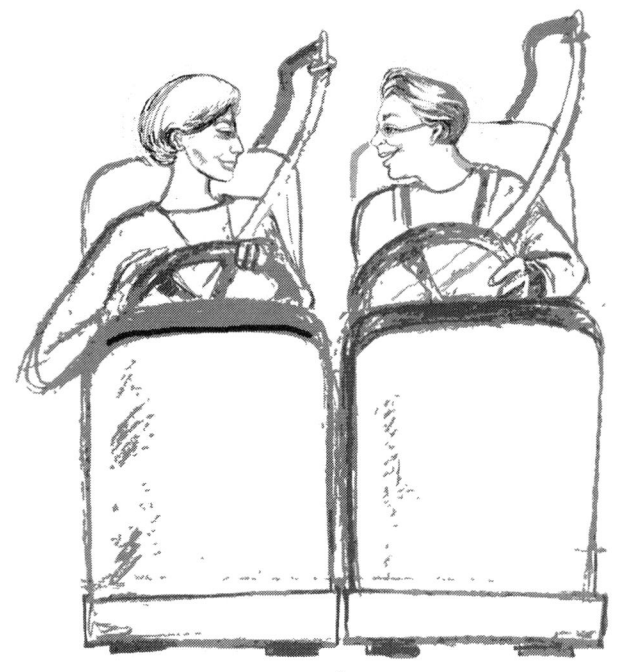

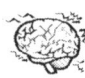 : Ready to try the stationary bike?

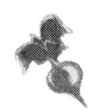 : Sure. And tomorrow–the pool!

Week 5

Walking Route

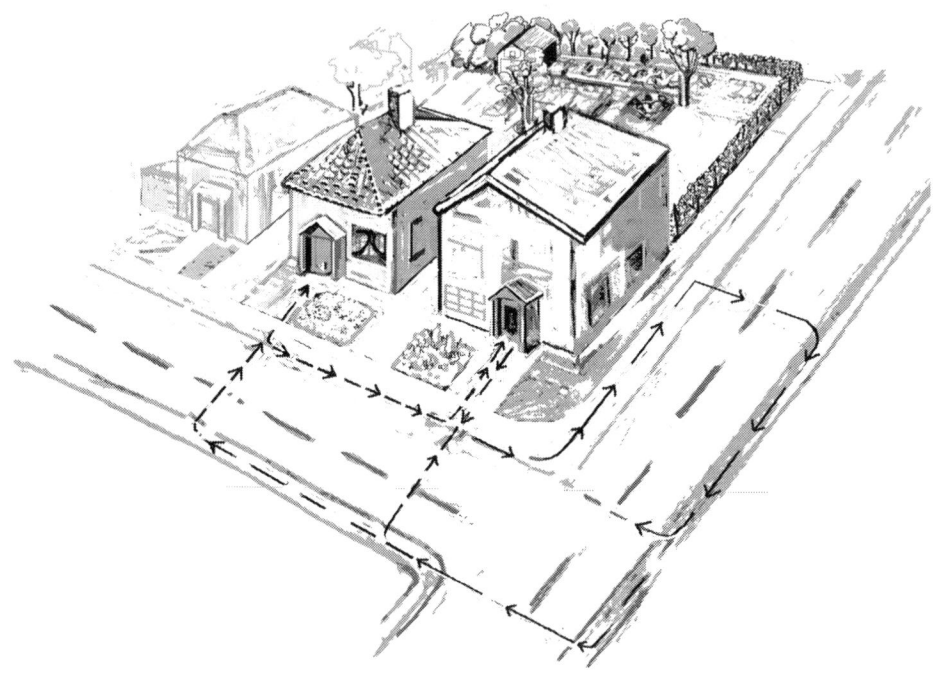

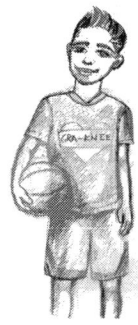

Jerome's Notes: The benefits of taking a circular route rather than walking directly out and back:

* Granny can cut her walk short if she needs to. She's never so far away that she has to walk in pain or beyond her endurance.

* She can adjust the length of the walk depending on how she feels, making the larger circle or the smaller circle.

* She can also mark her progress easily.

6 months

Happy Gardening

So that's pretty much it.

Granny graduated from Ms. Linda's class and her surgeon was really impressed with how quickly she progressed.

Now she walks for twenty minutes nearly every day, drives to the store to get her groceries, and catches the train to visit friends out of town.

She found a class where they practice movements like the ones Ms. Linda taught us and she goes every week.

Best of all, she is taking care of her garden again. She says she couldn't have done it all without me, and that I practice the best **TLA** there is—**TLC**.

Maybe when I grow up, I'll be a movement-learning specialist too.

May be.

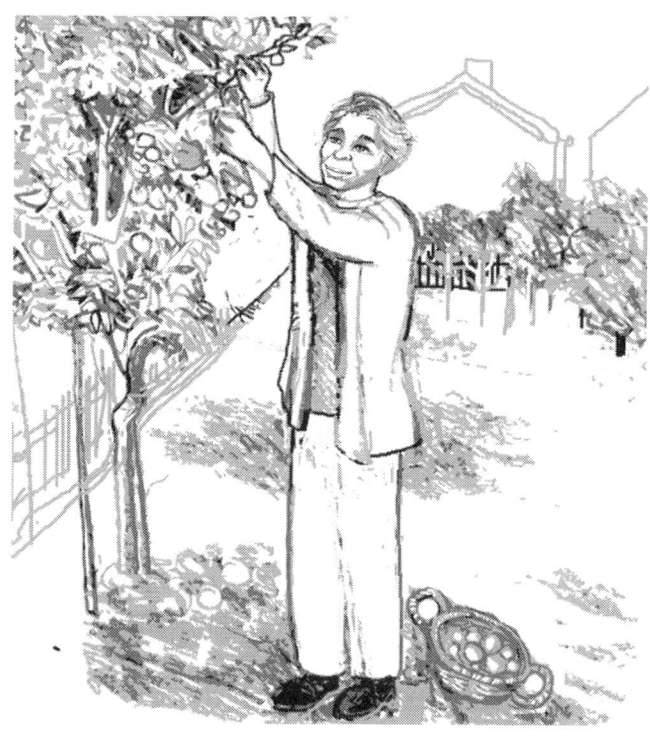

And a Whole Lot More

Handouts for Knee Replacement Preparation Classes

Compiled by Linda Thomas
Physical Therapist, Feldenkrais Teacher®

CONTENTS:

Before You Start	78
Pain and Ice and Elevation	80
Notes To Helpers	81
Improving Movement = Reducing Unnecessary Effort	83
Scanning Your Contact	84
The Lessons	86
Suggested Daily Schedule After Surgery:	
∗ In the Hospital	102
∗ At Home	104
Keys To Making Progress, Safely	106
The Big Picture	110
About Ms. Linda	117

The following handouts are intended to assist you in getting the most out of the Movement Lessons, which follow.

Please feel free to return to them often.

Before You Start

Location

Find a quiet place where you can be comfortable. A firm surface works best, but comfort is the top priority. Use pillows for support on the floor, a bed, or a flat wood chair. If turning to look to the side is painful when you are lying on your belly, prop yourself up on your forearms.

Slow, Small, Smooth

Make small movements slowly. As you improve the smoothness and ease of your movement, you can increase speed and size safely.

Do Less

Rather than pushing into or through the limit of the movement, sneak up on it. Be ready for your limits to change. If the instructions say, 'look towards the ceiling,' go only as far as you can in that direction, easily.

Reduce

Each time you practice a movement, reduce your effort.

Repetitions

The coordination of your whole self is key:

* Practice rather than repeat, so that your next movement is an improvement on the last

* Start with two or three of each movement in the sequence and leave it alone. The next day, review and progress, or do less if you experience any discomfort.

Remember, you are learning to move more freely in your daily life, not learning to do the lessons well.

Pausing

Taking a short pause between movements allows you to start a fresh movement without accumulated effort.

You also have an opportunity to digest what you learned from the previous movement.

Eyes Closed

Keeping eyes closed throughout each lesson reduces the distraction of 'creating' the external environment, and allows for easier attention to internal sensations.

Notice how your eyes move around to 'look' even when they are closed. They are making maps of your movement.

Both Sides

Practice the movements on both sides. This will reduce the differences in strength, flexibility, and coordination of the two legs in relation to your whole self. These differences can interfere with balance.

Hydration

Moving yourself differently can release toxins, which are best moved out by drinking lots of water.

PAIN is a sensation that tends to drown out all the other sensations. It demands attention. Seek immediate relief so that you can direct your attention to sensations of pressure, direction, speed, flow, and balance while practicing the lessons and moving through your day.

Coordinate with your healthcare professionals to find the best relief for you. Nothing is gained by gritting your teeth and braving it out.

If a movement increases pain, **STOP** and **REST**.

Make the movement again, smaller and slower. If it still hurts, practice on the other side, then come back to make one movement, or practice the movement by imagining the sequence, then make one movement. Do less, more often.

ICE can be applied to relieve pain before, during, or after practice of the movement lessons or after walking. You can use soft, moldable ice packs from the store, crushed ice in a wet towel, or frozen vegetables (rounded edges are best, like peas) in a towel. Wrap the ice around the whole joint for maximum relief.

Ask your healthcare providers to instruct you.

Use of ice for 15 – 20 minutes is effective in pain management, as it:

* Slows the speed of messages carried by the nerves, e.g. pain messages
* Reduces the energy demand of healing cells
* Restricts the blood flow, thereby reducing swelling

ELEVATION can help reduce swelling. Lie so that your feet are above your heart. If you sit up with your leg out on the couch, you can reduce the flow of blood back to your heart, like a kinked hose.

Notes to Helpers

Congratulations! You have in your heart the desire to support someone you love in their movement learning, and in your hands the means to safely guide them.

Your role is to read the lesson out loud, and to ask questions that direct attention to sensations.

Your 'Granny' will self-correct when s/he senses the difference between what s/he hears and intends to do, and what s/he is actually doing.

It takes patience to watch someone struggling to follow instructions.

Successful learning only requires sensing that your action is different from your intention and how—in size, speed, smoothness or direction.

Practice will lead to improvement for you both.

Let's look at an example of how this might work in a lesson.

In Helicopter Circles

You will offer the following **Instruction**:

* Please make small, slow, smooth circles in the air.

You may observe something other than this happening.

First, slowly repeat the instruction. If nothing changes, try asking the following Questions to direct attention to what is happening:

* Do your circles have edges?
* Are they the size of a volleyball? A tennis ball?

Then you can offer suggestions for **Redirecting**:

* Make the circle half as big
* Half as big again
* Half as fast
* Half as fast again

Or a combination of **Redirecting** and **Questions** to clarify what is different in the movements:

R: Make a circle moving only from the ankle. Now keep your ankle still and make a circle.

Q: Where does the movement come from? Does the pressure under your knee or hip change as you do this?

Improving Movement = Reducing Unnecessary Effort

When we attempt something new and unfamiliar, we often try too hard, making the movement jerky and unsatisfying. Notice any need to accomplish, and return your focus to sensations.

Be on the lookout for these signs of unnecessary effort:

* Clenched jaw
* Held breath
* Sudden jerky initiation of movement
* Clenched fists
* Fixed eyes or fast eye movements
  (These you can see under the closed eyelids)

If you see any of these happening, try asking the following Questions:

* Are your teeth touching?
* Are you breathing in or out as you begin the movement?
* Can you slowly build up to the needed effort to begin the movement?
* Are your hands soft and open?
* Are your closed eyes 'watching' the movement and matching its speed?

If the adjustment doesn't happen today, it may tomorrow, or the day after.

You are creating a learning environment — fun, rather than strict or demanding.

SCANNING YOUR CONTACT

Before you begin each lesson, lie down on your back on the floor or a firm bed, and close your eyes. Notice where you make contact and where you don't. You can start with the back of your head, moving down your spine to your shoulder blades and arms, continuing down your spine, out to your ribs, to your low back, sacrum, pelvis, hips, backs of your knees, calves and heels. Comparing right and left sides, noticing how your breathing changes your contact, and what your eyes are doing throughout.

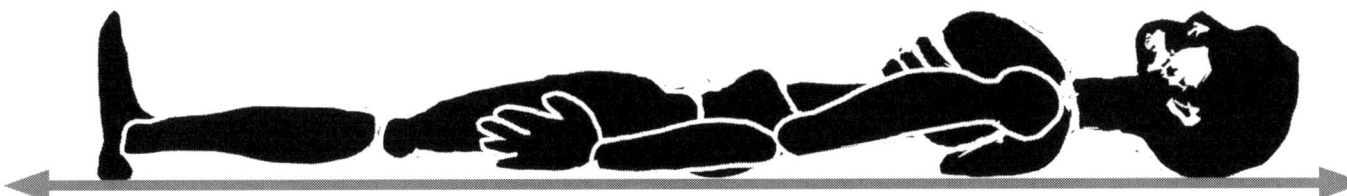

Remember this contact scan so you can compare it with your contact scans during and after each lesson practice. You can return to lying on your back to scan your contact during a **PAUSE** or **REST**. For the sitting and standing lessons, you can scan the contact of your pelvis and feet when you **PAUSE** in the lesson.

As you practice scanning your contact each day, your accuracy in sensing differences will improve. You will also be able to track how you are responding to the lessons.

Lesson 1

SOFT SHOE SHUFFLE PRIMER

Sit towards the front of a hard, flat chair with no arms.

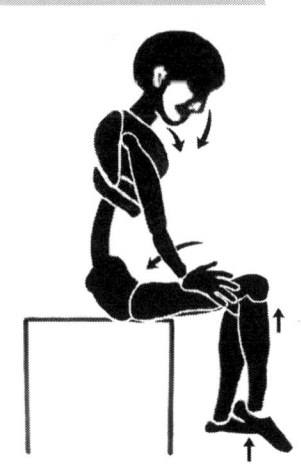

A: Lift your **(R)** heel up and down. Notice that your **(R)** knee goes up and down with your heel and the angle of your **(R)** hip closes and opens. Move slowly in order to sense what you are doing. **PAUSE** after each up and down.

B: Look towards your belly button as you roll back on your pelvis and lift your **(R)** heel. Then look towards the ceiling as you roll forward on your pelvis and lower your **(R)** heel. **PAUSE. PRACTICE** breathing out as you fold, breathing in as you lengthen and look up.

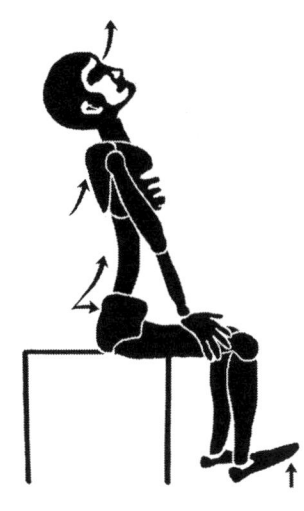

C: Continue folding and lengthening, and begin to rock back on your heel, lifting your toes as you look up, lowering toes and lifting heel as you look to your belly button. **PAUSE**.

D: Now **PRACTICE** a different combination of folding and lengthening. Look up as you lift your heel up and roll your pelvis back, then lower your heel and lift your toes up as you roll your pelvis forward and look to your belly button. **REST. PRACTICE** moving continuously between the two movements as you breathe out and in, in and out.

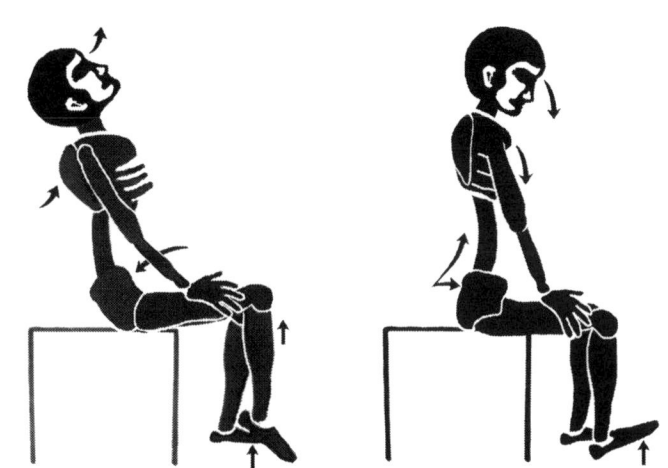

86 · Granny Gets a New Knee

Slide your **(R)** foot in Soft Shoe Shuffle then your **(L)** foot.

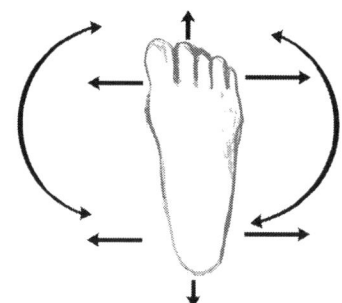

* Does one foot/leg move more easily?
  Is one leg lighter?

Stand up and walk around.

Compare the sensations of contact each foot is making with the floor.

E: Sit again and **PRACTICE** with **(L)** heel/toes.

Keeping it fresh: Lift your heel up and lower it a little to the Right, lift again and return to starting position. **PAUSE**. Lift your heel and lower it a little to the Left, lift again and return to the starting position.

Lesson 2
TWIST AGAIN

Lie on your **(L)** side, knees bent comfortably, **(R)** on top of **(L)**, pillows between your knees and feet and under your head, **(L)** arm directly in front of you with your **(R)** elbow above your **(R)** hand which rests somewhere near your **(L)** elbow. Eyes closed.

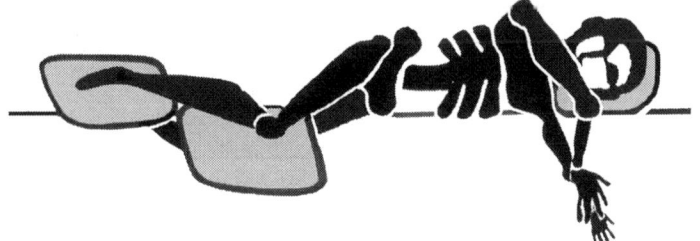

A: Bring your **(R)** knee away from your **(L)** knee and back, keeping your feet together. **PAUSE. PRACTICE** this a few times. Now add rolling your head to 'look' right towards the ceiling and back,

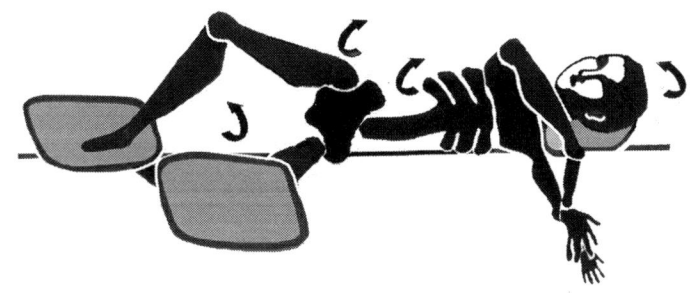

as you lift your knee away and back. **PAUSE** after each movement away and back. Move **SLOWLY**.

*   Does your underside leg change contact as you lift and lower your knee?

*   Do you breathe out or in as you lift your knee? Try both ways.

*   Can you free your ribs and shoulder blades to allow your arms to stay still?

B: Tilt your **(R)** leg to bring your **(R)** foot away from your **(L)** foot and back, keeping your knees together. **PAUSE**. **PRACTICE** this a few times. Now add rolling your head to 'look' left towards the floor and back, as you lift and lower your foot. **PAUSE** after each movement.

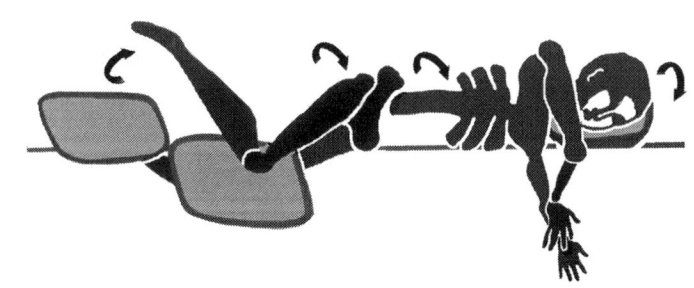

88 · Granny Gets a New Knee

* Do you breathe out or in as you lift your foot? Try both ways.

* Does your pelvis roll forward and back with your knee and foot?

* Do your ribs come together and away? Do they push into the floor or bed?

C: Now **PRACTICE** a different combination. Turn to 'look' right as you lift your foot, then return to look forward as you lower your foot. **PAUSE** after each movement. Move **SLOWLY**. **PRACTICE**.

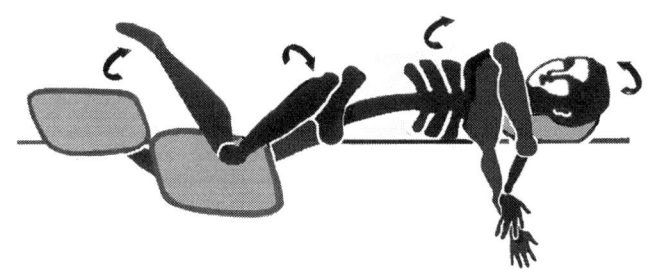

D: Turn to 'look' left as you lift your knee, then return to look forward as you lower your knee. **PAUSE** after each movement. **PRACTICE**.

E: Now move between **A** and **B** in a continuous motion, moving to match your breathing in and out. **PAUSE**. Now move between **C** and **D**. **REST**.

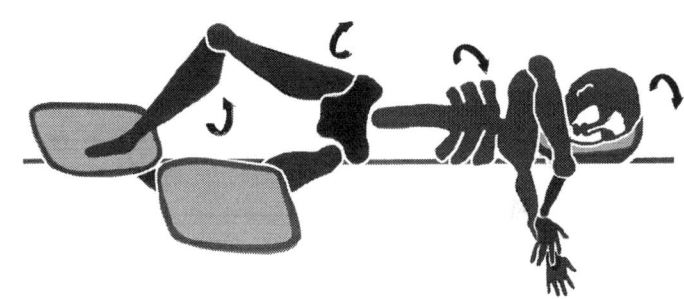

Stand up **SLOWLY** and walk around. Look to right and left.

* Is one way easier?

F: Lie down on your **(R)** side and go through the 'mirror' sequence, substituting **(L)** for **(R)** and **(R)** for **(L)**.

Stand up **SLOWLY** and walk around. You might sense yourself as taller, longer in the front, lighter in the legs, or more flexible in the middle.

Granny Gets a New Knee

Lesson 3
HELICOPTER CIRCLES

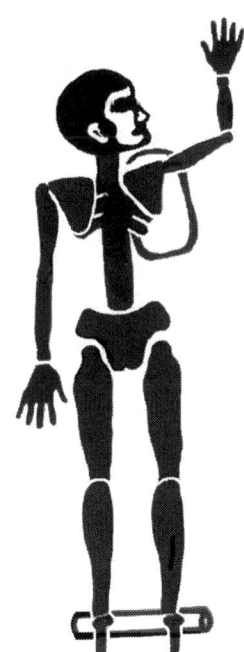

Lie on your belly, head turned to the Right, pillow under your **(R)** shoulder, rolled up towel under your ankles. Eyes closed.

If you experience contact pain in your knee, place a flat cushion under your thigh to 'float' your knee when you bend. If you are uncomfortable turning your head to the side, prop yourself up on your forearms.

A: Bend your **(L)** knee to lift your **(L)** foot off the towel an inch or two and lower it. Start very **SLOWLY. PRACTICE, PAUSING** after each lift and lower.

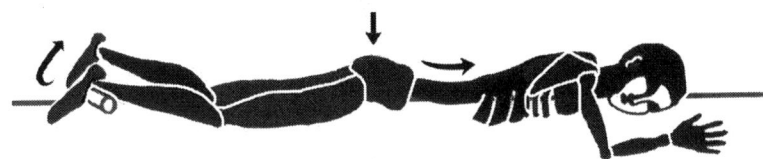

* Does your **(L)** hip move towards or away from the floor?

* Do you need to tense your calf muscle to lift your foot? Or is bending your knee sufficient? Place your **(L)** hand under your **(L)** hip, palm up, to help sense this.

B: Now bring your **(L)** foot up over your **(L)** knee, then lower your **(L)** foot to the left of you, and back up. One time let your toes go out first, then let your heel go out first, rotating your lower leg. **PAUSE. PRACTICE.**

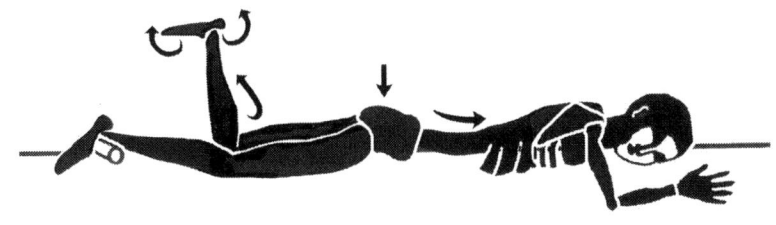

* Do you effort to turn your lower leg? Or let go?

Return to the towel and **REST**. Lift and turn your head to the left and return to face to the right. Move very **SLOWLY** to ease any stiffness in your neck.

C: Bring your **(L)** foot over your knee again, lower your foot out to the left and make small, slow, smooth circles in the air. **PAUSE**. Change the direction of the circles. **REST** whenever you fatigue, either in muscles or attention.

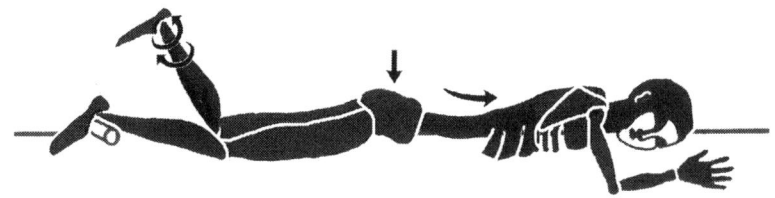

Bend both knees then tilt both feet all the way to the left picking up your knees and pelvis to roll you onto your back. **REST**.

* Does one leg lie closer to the bed? Is one leg longer? Lighter?

D: Roll to lie on your belly again. Switch the position of your arms and turn your head to look left. **PRACTICE** with your **(R)** foot.

Keeping it fresh – lower your foot towards the other leg, change the angle of your knee, make circles, figure of 8's, other numbers, or letters of the alphabet.

Lesson 4

CLIMBING THE WALLS

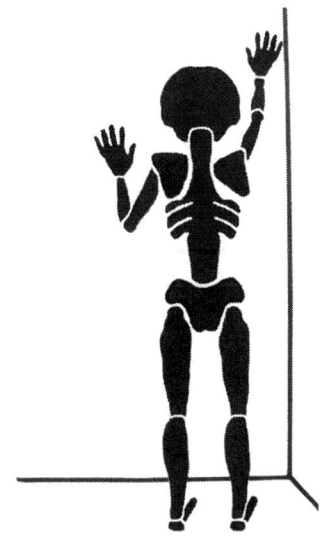

Stand one long step away from a vacant wall with your **(L)** palm on the wall at shoulder height and your **(R)** palm a little higher.

A: Take a step forward with your **(R)** foot, allowing your **(R)** hand to slide up the wall comfortably. Your **(L)** heel will rise through a soft **(L)** knee as you shift your weight over your **(R)** leg. Keeping your **(R)** foot where it is, lengthen your **(L)** heel to the floor without bending your **(L)** knee, sliding your **(R)** hand down the wall. **(L)** hand stays in place throughout, **(R)** knee will bend a little as your **(L)** heel lowers. **PAUSE**.

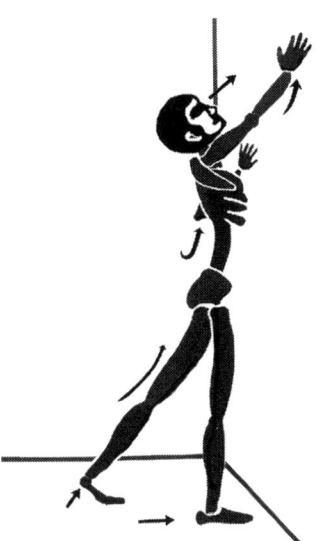

PRACTICE several times, looking at your **(R)** hand sliding up as you rock forward, returning to look directly ahead as your heel lengthens to the floor.

B: With your hands in the same position as for **A**, your **(R)** foot forward and your **(L)** foot back a little, lift your **(L)** heel as you fold to look at your bending **(L)** knee, then lower your **(L)** heel to the floor as you return to looking forward. **PAUSE**. **PRACTICE** a few times. Now add in sliding your **(R)** hand down the wall as you fold to look at your bending **(L)** knee, and look up at your **(R)** hand sliding up the wall as your **(L)** heel lowers to the floor.

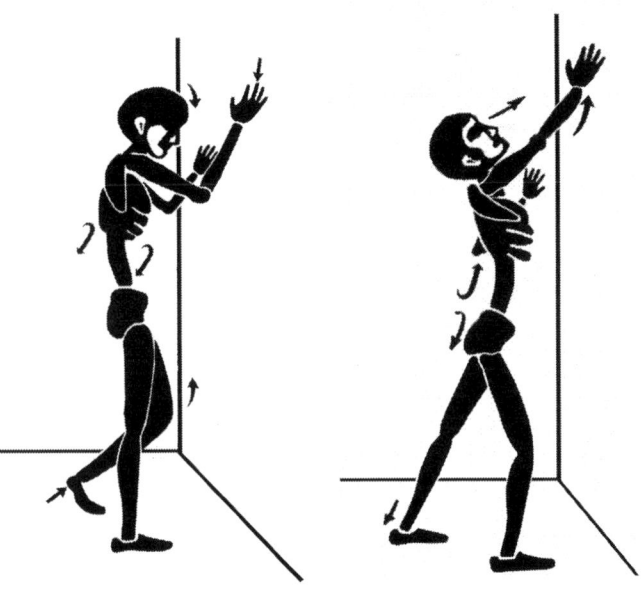

92 · *Granny Gets a New Knee*

PAUSE. PRACTICE several times, breathing out as you look down, breathing in as you look up. Walk around a little.

* Is there a difference in your stride length or push off **(L)** to **(R)**?

This sequence can be **PRACTICED** after surgery while standing with your hands on your walker. Walk around and sense how your pelvis moves over your foot and beyond.

C: Return to the wall, and with hands in the same positions, look left as you lift your **(L)** heel through a soft **(L)** knee, sliding your **(R)** hand up. As you return, leading through your **(L)** heel with **(R)** hand sliding down the wall, look forward. **PAUSE. PRACTICE**.

* How easily does your **(R)** hand slide up the wall now compared to when you started?

Walk around a little.

* Are you longer in the front? Eyes focused differently? Torso moving around? Head freer?

D: Return to the wall and **PRACTICE** pushing off and lowering through your **(R)** heel and knee, sliding your **(L)** hand up and down, following instructions for **A**, **B**, and **C**.

Lesson 5

FIRST MOVEMENTS

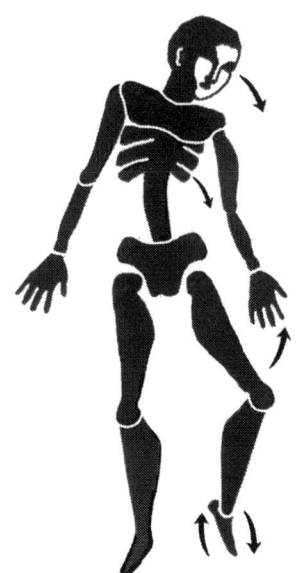

Lie on your back, legs long, eyes closed.

A: At the same time, **SLOWLY** roll your non-op leg out to the side, bending your knee **AND** turn to look toward the bending side. Return to looking forward as you lengthen your leg. **PAUSE**. **PRACTICE**.

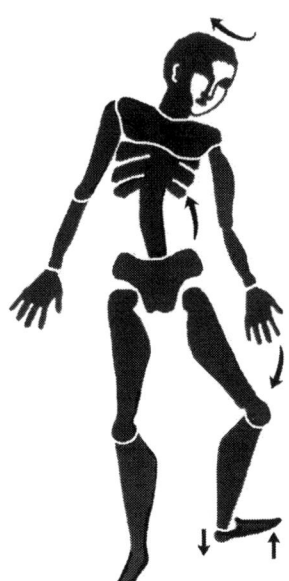

B: Turn to look at your bending side, pointing your toes as you bend, then pushing your heel away as you lengthen your leg and look forward. Now push your heel away as you bend, then point your toes as you lengthen. **PAUSE. PRACTICE**.

* Does your whole spine roll with your hip and head? Bringing your ribs on one side closer to the bed?

C: Roll the same hip out and up to stand on your foot. Separate your standing foot and long leg from each other and begin to lower your 'standing' knee towards your 'new' knee, breathing in. Breathe out as you raise your knee back up. Do this several times, **PAUSING** between each movement, softening your spine, ribs, and jaw.

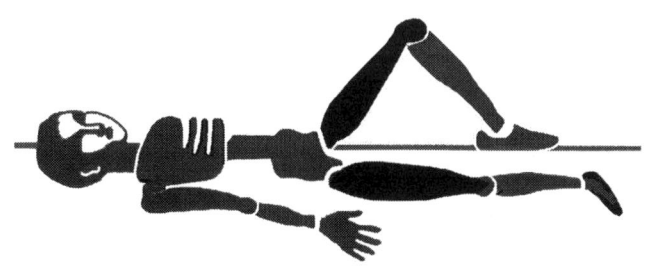

* Does your pelvis follow your knee? Does your head follow your pelvis?

D: Begin to lengthen through your knee as you lower it, so that your pelvis rolls and turns your other leg out, and your head rolls too. Return. As you **PRACTICE**, allow this movement to grow to include drawing your 'new' knee up a little, then lengthen your 'operated side' leg as your hip, pelvis and head return.

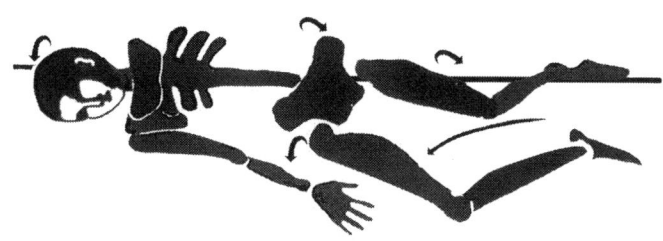

PRACTICE these movements for 3-5 minutes every 15-20 minutes when you wake up after surgery.

Lesson 6

THE FLOOR IS MY FRIEND

Sit on the front edge of a sofa, bed or seat with space to the right of you. It is best to find a surface where your hips are higher than your knees. As you progress, a lower surface will be more challenging.

A: Begin sliding your **(R)** hand to the right and back. **PAUSE.** Now look at your hand as you slide away and return to look forward as you slide back. **PAUSE. PRACTICE** this movement, breathing in as you turn to look right, out as you look forward.

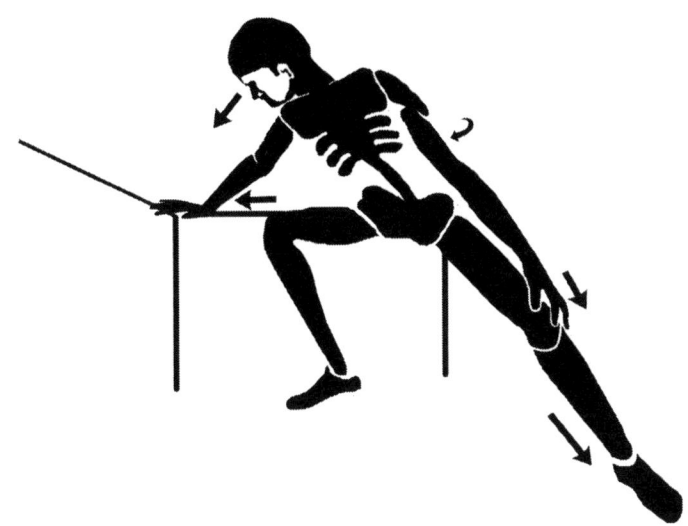

* Which hip does your weight shift over?

Continue sliding your **(R)** hand away and turning your head to the right, and add sliding your **(L)** foot out in front of you, lengthening your **(L)** leg. Slide your **(L)** foot back as you slide your hand back and look forward. **PAUSE. PRACTICE** this movement, breathing out as you turn to look right, in as you look forward. **REST**.

Now add sliding your **(L)** hand down your lengthening **(L)** leg and back as you return your leg and **(R)** hand. Your hands will be moving away from each other and back towards each other with each movement. **PAUSE. PRACTICE** this so that the movements of your hands and leg away and back start and finish at the same time.

B: The next time you lengthen and slide away, stay there and bring your **(L)** hand to rest flat on the floor about halfway between your feet. If you can't reach the floor, use a short stool under your **(L)** hand. Now begin to lean forward and lower your head. As your head goes down, notice how the weight on your pelvis is lightening. Find the balance point where your head goes down and your pelvis can slide to the left and lift up a little. Try changing the position of your hands to help you push up. Return your pelvis to sit. Then bring your head all the way up. **PAUSE. PRACTICE** one to two movements, over many days, sliding with your **(L)** hand to the left and lengthening your **(R)** leg, before proceeding.

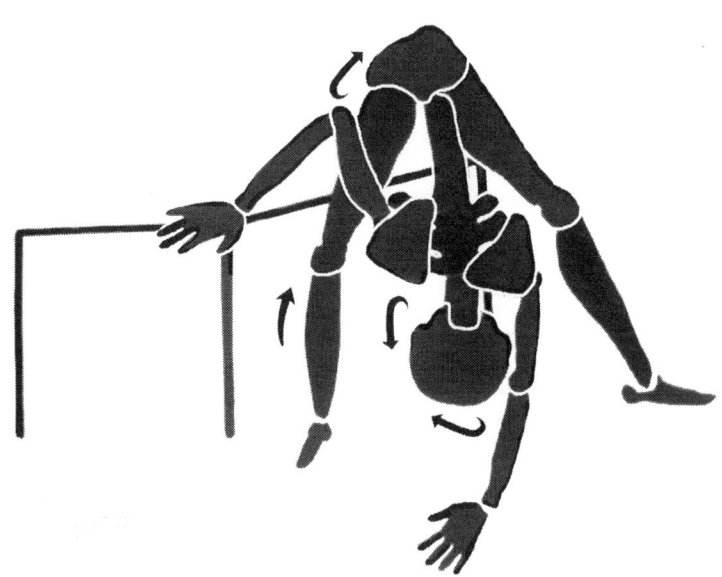

C: Lower your head to lift your pelvis away from the seat as for **B**, now look over your **(R)** foot and swivel your **(L)** foot so that you can begin to lower your **(L)** knee towards the floor. This is like the start position in a running race. Bring your knee up and swivel to sit again. **PAUSE. PRACTICE** a few movements over a few days on both sides.

You do not need to go through the whole sequence for this lesson to improve your relationship with the floor. When you can breathe throughout the sequence and easily reach the floor, continue.

Return to your runner's start position and begin to lightly touch your **(L)** knee to the floor, then to the floor a little to the right and then a little to the left. Return to sitting whenever needed.

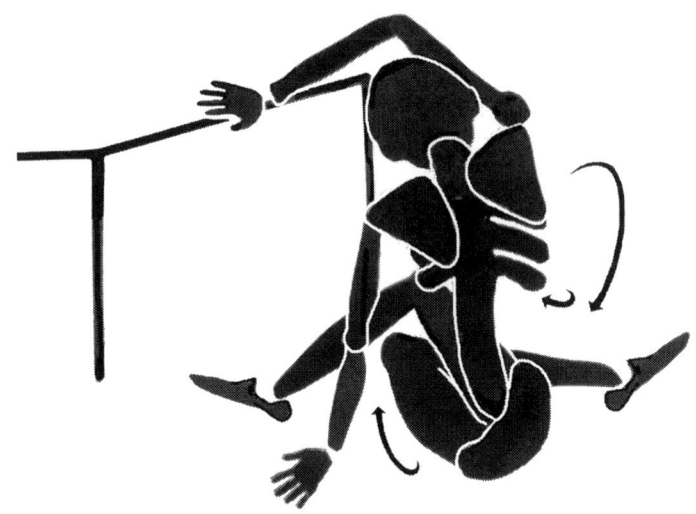

Next time you move your **(L)** knee to the right, begin to look over your **(R)** shoulder, and return to your running start. **PAUSE**. **PRACTICE** this movement several times, looking over your **(R)** shoulder, gradually sliding your **(L)** knee further to the right, allowing your pelvis to follow towards the floor. Return to your runner's start position, then lift your **(L)** knee up and return your pelvis to sitting. **REST**.

Take several days to lower your **(L)** knee and pelvis closer to the floor and back up, only going so far as you can reverse the movement easily and breathe in both directions. Make only a few movements on each side, and walk around. You may find it easier to touch the floor with your **(R)** knee. Respect your limits on each side.

D: When you can attend to your breathing as you move, put **A B C** together, moving from seat to the floor and back, and continue to practice once every other day.

JUST FOR FUN

On the next two pages, you will find a movement sequence made by connecting parts of the Six Lessons you have already practiced. The key tells you which part of each Lesson is used.

Take a peek and see if you recognize the movements.

Now, **PRACTICE** moving back and forth between a few movements at a time, **SLOWLY**. Then, **PRACTICE** putting together the entire sequence in both directions.

Move fluidly, without holding your breath. Find your grace and ease.

1. *Climbing the Walls:* **A**

2. *Breathing Down*

3. *The Floor Is My Friend:* **A**-hand sliding, head and torso following until legs lift, like a teeter-totter

4. *Twist Again:* **A**

5. *First Movements:* **D**

6. *Twist Again:* **B**

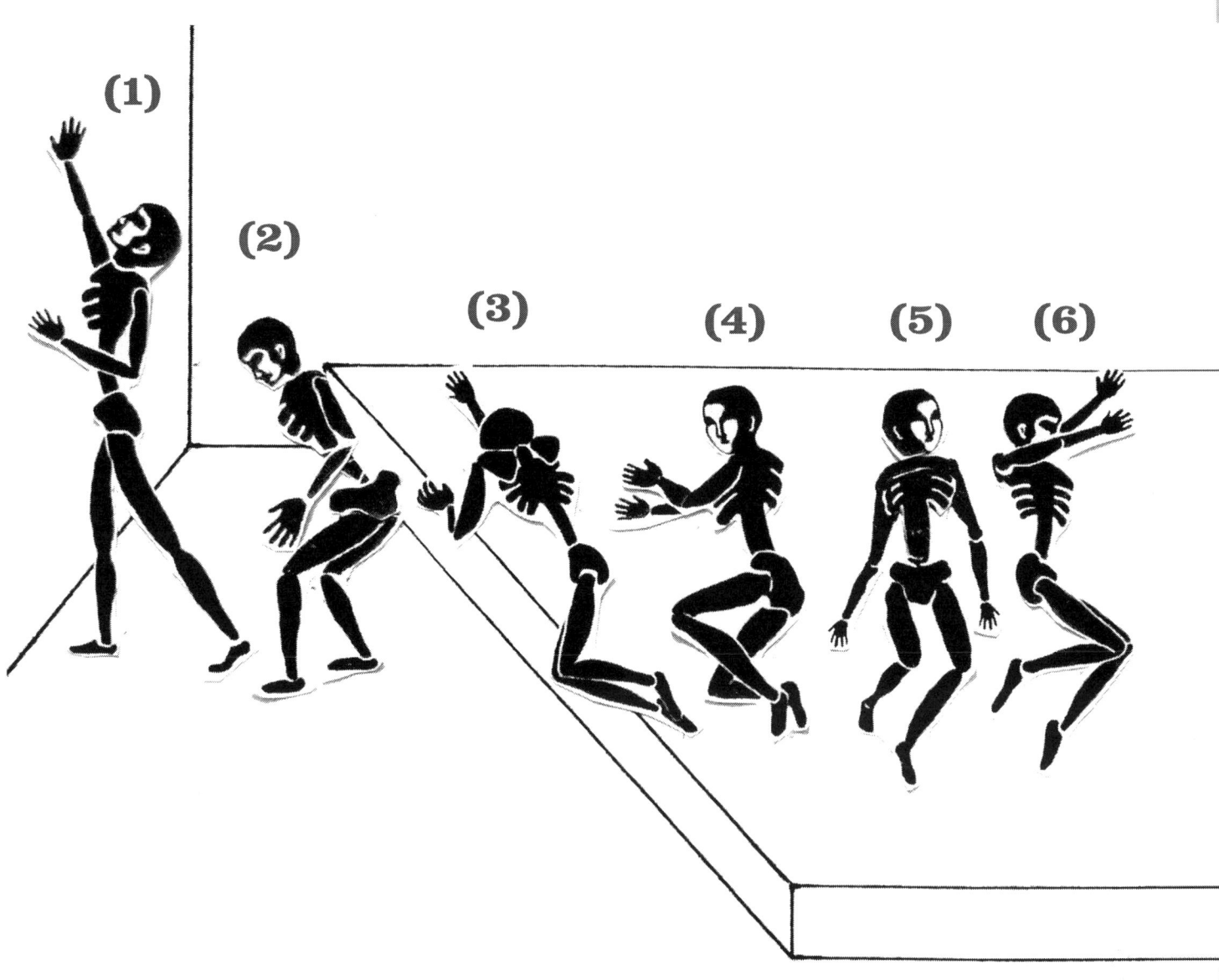

100 · Granny Gets a New Knee

7. *Helicopter Circles:* **B**

8. *Helicopter Circles:* **B**-both legs lower to the same side together

9. Continue to lower your feet over the edge towards the floor, spiraling your pelvis, torso and finally head

10. *Soft Shoe Shuffle Primer:* **B**

11. Imagine yourself here: *Breathing Up*

12. *Climbing The Walls:* **A**

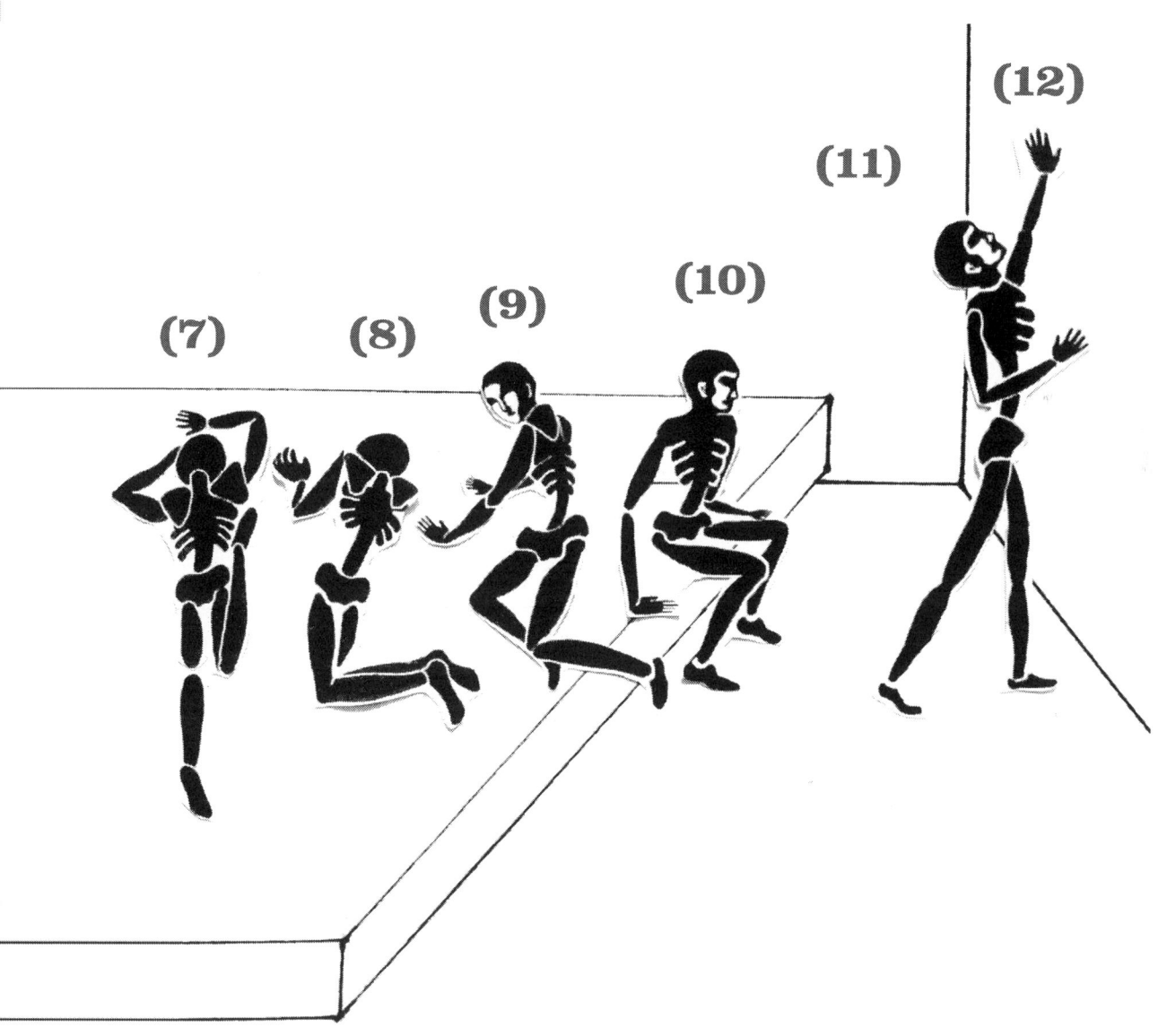

Suggested Daily Schedule after Surgery:

In the Hospital

1. As soon as you wake up after the surgery, begin to imagine your *First Movements* on your non-operated side, continuing through the full sequence. Notice how your closed eyes shift between the two sides, and begin to grow micro-movements with your eyes and breathing on the operated side. Pause often. Continue growing the movements, bringing in your pelvis and spine. Focus on coordinating your whole self rather than making large movements. Remember to separate your legs to allow your standing knee space to lower towards your operated knee. Practice a few movements every 15–20 minutes.

2. You will be encouraged to pump your ankles for circulation. Think of lengthening through your heels, then lengthening through your toes, as you do in the *First Movements* sequence. Move slowly at first, and then make small, quick movements so that you slide up and down through your whole self against the bed. Your chin will come closer to your chest when you lengthen through your toes, away from your chest when you lengthen through your heels. Alternate your movements so that one side is lengthening through your heel while the other side is lengthening through your toes, back and forth. Practice a few movements every 15–20 minutes.

3. Roll to your non-operated side and begin your *Twist Again* sequence. Imagining first, then micro-movements with your eyes and breathing, progressing to a few movements, twice a day.

4. Hospital staff will assist you to sit when you are medically stable. Practice a few *Soft Shoe Shuffle* movements at the side of the bed before standing up and walking. Adjust the height of your bed as needed for standing up (try a little higher) and sitting down (try a little lower).

5. Imagine rolling from your back to your side to your belly as in the *Just For Fun* sequence. Imagine moving through your *Helicopter Circles* sequence. You will begin to practice these movements once you are at home. Remember to use a flat pillow under your thigh to float your knee.

Suggested Daily Schedule after Surgery:

At Home

When you wake up – in bed:
* *First Movements* – 5 minutes, then sit up
* *Soft Shoe Shuffle* or *Primer* – 5 minutes, then stand up
* Short walk

Mid-Late Morning
* *Climbing the Walls* – 5 minutes
* Climbing up and down stairs inside or outside and/or short walk

Mid Afternoon – lying on bed:
* *Twist Again* and/or *Helicopter Circles*, 10 minutes, then
* **REST** with Ice, with feet elevated above heart if swelling, then
* *First Movements* and/or *Soft Shoe Shuffle Primer* – 10 minutes, then
* Short walk

End of Day – in bed:
* *First Movements* – 5 minutes

During the Night – before or after using bathroom/fetching ice:

* *First Movements*, or whichever lesson helps reduce pain, then
* *Soft Shoe Shuffle*

Every other Day, or Several Times a Week:

* *The Floor is My Friend* - this challenging sequence provides an opportunity to improve your strength, balance, and coordination.

Keys to Making Progress, Safely

KEEP MOVING

If you stay still in one position for longer than an hour or so, you will tend towards stiffness. Change your position frequently and walk around throughout the day, slowly increasing your distance.

FOR EVERY 20 MINUTES OF SITTING:

Soft Shoe Shuffle for 3 – 5 minutes, then take a short walk. If you tend to lose track of time sitting at the computer or reading, set an alarm and get up to walk around. Better to sit for several shorter sessions than one long one.

STANDING

If you need to stand for longer than a few minutes for any reason, move your feet around, shifting your weight side to side, and forward and back. Walk around a little, and come back.

TRANSITIONS

ROLLING OVER

To roll from your side to your back, practice the Twist Again movements where you look towards the ceiling while lifting your knee, then continue slowly until your pelvis, spine, and head roll all the way over.

To roll from your back to your side, practice the First Movements, continuing to lengthen your knee and turn your pelvis, bringing the whole spine and head over the other side.

To roll onto your belly from your side, practice the Twist Again movements where you look towards the floor while lifting your foot, continuing all the way over, bringing your arm under you or around the top of your head.

LYING TO SITTING

Lie on your back, lengthening through your knee as in First Movements, bringing your head closer to your knees and making yourself into a ball. Then, lower your legs off the side, pushing up to sitting.

OR

Lie on your side and tilt both feet up as in the Twist Again sequence, lowering them towards the floor as your torso comes up, like a corkscrew teeter totter.

SITTING TO LYING

Begin to slide your hand towards the head of the bed, watching your hand, as your torso lengthens against the bed to follow your hand. As the balance of your weight shifts through your pelvis towards your sliding hand, the top side of your torso shortens, and lifts your legs.

SIT TO STAND

After practicing any of the lessons, sit for a moment and look up and down a few times, rolling your pelvis forward and back in time with your in and out breath. When you are ready to stand up, lead with your eyes—SEE where you are going breathing in, rolling your pelvis forward, and continuing up over your feet in a fluid motion towards your destination. If needed, use your hands to push yourself up before bringing them up to the walker, crutch or cane.

STAND TO SIT

Stand with the back of your non-surgical knee against the chair or bed. Breathe out as you fold yourself into your pelvis, sliding your surgical leg away. Think of your eyes leading through your tail. If needed, reach back with both hands to support your weight as you lower yourself to sit.

WALKING

As you walk, your muscles contract and relax, acting as a pump to circulate your blood which carries fresh oxygen and nutrients to every cell. After the lessons, attentive, slow walking gives you an opportunity to notice how your practice carries over into your everyday activities.

WALKING BACKWARDS

Turn around inside your walker so that the horizontal bar is behind you. You will be pushing your walker backwards too. Make sure you have a clear space behind you with no obstacles, and have someone watch you the first time. Slide the ball of your foot back along the floor keeping your knee straight. Lead through your heel as you do in Climbing The Walls, and rock your weight back on this foot. Then, do the same with the other side. Imagine your eyes are on the back of your head, 'looking' where you are going.

STAIRS

It will boost your confidence to have someone 'spot' you when you begin to go up and down stairs–just like rock climbers!

Practice going up and down 2 steps one day, then next day 2 steps once in the morning, once in the afternoon, then next day 2 steps in the morning, 3 steps in the afternoon, gradually adding as long as there is no increase in pain or swelling while you are doing it or several hours later. At first you will go up with your non-surgical side leading.

Practice bending your hip and knee to gently place your surgical side foot on the lowest step and back down at least once every day. Over several weeks, you will begin to gently lean forward AS IF to step up on this side. Remember to look where you are going–UP.

Practice backing down the stairs while you face the top of the stairs, leading with your heel the way you do in the Climbing The Walls lesson.

The Big Picture

BREATHING

The breathing lesson on page 61, like the other lessons, is intended to focus attention on the sensations generated by specific movements in specific positions. It will help you sense your breathing in relation to your moving, improving both.

Here are some factors that influence when, how often, and how deeply you breathe:

* The need to blow off a build-up of carbon dioxide or CO_2, which in high concentrations is poisonous. (It is the blood level of CO_2 that triggers the brain to breathe)

* Your level of activity. How much CO_2 is produced when oxygen or O_2 is used to produce energy, determines how often, and how deeply you breathe. (O_2 + glucose = CO_2 + water + energy)

* Volume and pressure of airflow required for level of vocal expression. (It is higher for singing or yelling than speaking)

* The flexibility of the ribs and spine in all directions. (The largest lung capacity is in the lower lobes, which are in the back of you–out of sight, brought into mind by attention to the sensations of movement in the ribs, breast bone, belly, and back with breathing)

* The softness of the belly and low back when the diaphragm flattens and drops, drawing air in.

* The changing configuration of the skeleton during activities, e.g. when lying on your back it is harder for air to enter the lower lobes, when you are crouched down or fearful, the belly is compressed.

THE TWO ELEPHANTS IN THE ROOM

GRAVITY – The mass of planet Earth is constantly pulling us towards it. Our every movement is in relation to this gravitational pull. We exert muscular effort to configure our skeleton for movement away from, across, and towards the planet. Our huge brains organize how we do this throughout our lives. We can listen to this via our senses as it happens, playing with infinite possibilities, or move on autopilot.

TIME – is not a commodity. It cannot be spent, wasted, saved, or expired. It has no location. It cannot fly, crawl, gallop, or stand still. Listening to sensations provoked by movement can be an experience of timelessness–a daily gift I hope you will give yourself.

RESTING

I cannot say enough about the merits of the mid afternoon, or midmorning **REST**.

Sink into your quiet self, then return to upright life, refreshed and ready.

You may or may not sleep. It doesn't matter.

Call it a power nap, snooze, rest, or siesta – whatever works.

Just **TRY IT**.

EQUIPMENT LIST

Order what you need from this list so they can be delivered a few days before surgery and you can practice using them.

Ice Packs – two large, flexible ice packs so you can rotate them, or multiple bags of large frozen peas

Walker – wheeled or pick up depending on your home terrain and how much you will be leaning on it–ask.

Crutches – allow you to move faster, and to go up stairs. Graduating to one crutch frees up one hand for carrying things.

Cane – when you need only a little support and also to signal to others to be careful when passing you.

Walking Poles – when you are ready to increase your cardiovascular endurance, and to assist in the rhythm of your stride.

Commode – with arm rests for over the toilet, or for use at bedside. Using a commode allows you to sit and stand without having to bend down as far.

Shower stool – in tub-shower or stall.

Handheld Shower Head – gives you control of the water while sitting on the stool in the tub-shower or stall.

Reacher – for picking things up off the floor.

Long shoe horn – enables you to wear shoes with a back.

Wedge and Back support – for the car. Sit on the wedge with your pelvis all the way back to create a more level surface, and use the back support to fill the gap between you and the car seat back. This reduces the effort in your thigh muscles and promotes the natural curves in your spine to support your head and enable freer turning for safer driving.

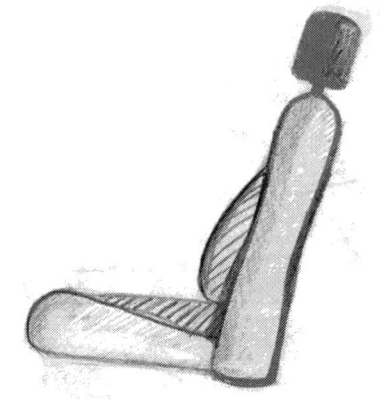

FREQUENTLY ASKED QUESTIONS

Q: I don't have a bathroom downstairs, and I don't think I'll be able to go up the stairs when I first get home. What should I do?

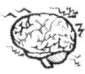 : You can use the commode with the bucket in place for toileting, and soapy washcloths and a bowl of warm water for bathing basics. You can practice going up and down a few stairs several times a day without the pressure of having to get all the way up or down, building up to the reward of a nice hot shower after your staples have been removed.

Q: I get up to go to the bathroom a lot in the night. I am concerned about using the walking equipment safely when I get around.

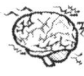 : The commode with the bucket in place can be kept by the bed at night and emptied and replaced over the toilet by a caregiver in the morning. You can also put in a nightlight, or have a lamp within easy reach of the bed.

Q: Do I have to remove all the area rugs?

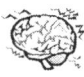 : In the first days and sometimes weeks after surgery you may be taking medicines that can affect your focus. You want to reduce the chances of catching your walker, crutches, cane, or toe and a potential fall. You can do this by removing small, thin rugs in all living areas, bedroom and bathrooms. It is worth the effort, and often gives you a longer stretch of open 'road' to practice your walking. Alternatively, you can tape down the edges or use anti-slip pads under your rugs.

Q: **I live alone, but I have family and friends in the area who have offered to help. How much help will I need when I come home after the surgery?**

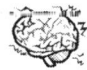 : Everyone's recovery is different, but in the first 2 – 3 weeks at least, I think it is better to set up a lot of help rather than overdoing it yourself and lengthening your healing process. Think about your daily needs:

* Meals – Have someone shop for your basic supplies and ask family/friends to drop off your favorite healthy dishes, which can be stretched to last 2 meals. You can start preparing one simple meal per day after 2 weeks if you are comfortable weight-bearing for 20 – 30 minutes.

* When using a walker or two crutches, you will not be able to carry a cup, bowl, or plate. Having someone around at meal times is helpful.

* Hopefully you have practiced getting into your shower or bath using your equipment, and the visiting healthcare staff will check that with you. If you are not completely comfortable, it is good to have someone present the first couple of times until you are confident.

* While it is not essential to have someone go through the lessons with you each day, another person can keep you on schedule, encourage, and support you. They can fetch and carry ice from the freezer as well.

Q: How do I know when it is time to progress from the walker through the crutches to the cane?

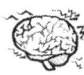 : The most important thing is to use the level of support you need in any given moment. The walker provides the greatest stability, and keeps you moving slowly. As you gain confidence, and begin to walk more easily, the walker will feel less like a necessity and more like a nuisance. Try the crutches and the walker for a few days, then just the crutches. Start using one crutch after your lesson practice, knowing you can use both crutches if needed. You are ready to graduate to a cane or no device when you find you have left the crutch somewhere without thinking about it. The cane is used primarily for balance and, when you are out in the world, to let people know they should move around you with care.

Note: If you have stairs with a handrail, you will want to keep a crutch nearby to use when going up and down. No handrail? Use both crutches.

Q: How long do I need to keep doing the suggested daily schedule?

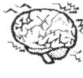 : The first two to six months after surgery are key to your long-term mobility. If you take this time to integrate your new knee components: moving through your schedule every day, progressing your daily walking and stair climbing, listening to your needs for rest, movement, and pain relief, you will reap the full benefits of your surgery.

Q: I just found 'Granny' and my surgery is next week. What should I do?

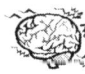 : Breathe. Organize your support system. Begin learning the lessons, one each day and practicing the lesson from the previous day, building up to the Suggested Daily Schedule on page 104. The essential lessons are Soft Shoe Shuffle Primer, Twist Again, Helicopter Circles, and First Movements. You can add in Climbing the Walls and The Floor is My Friend after the surgery. Move slowly so you can be inside your movements. Rushing through the lessons will not serve you.

Q: How do I find someone who teaches movement like Ms. Linda?

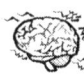 : Go to *http://feldenkrais.com* or ask someone you know to do this if you don't have access to a computer. Ms. Linda is a Feldenkrais Teacher.

Ms. Linda Thomas, PT, FT

Linda Thomas trained first as a Physical Therapist, then as a Feldenkrais Teacher. She has worked in hospitals, home health, professional clinics and private practice, on three continents. Ms. Linda now shares her 30+ years of movement learning and teaching experience with her students.

Her Motto: No Pain, Great Gain.

The Feldenkrais Method® of Somatic Education

Simply put – it is body learning through focused attention to differences in sensation as we move.

The Feldenkrais Method is practiced in two ways:

FUNCTIONAL INTEGRATION®

A Feldenkrais Teacher uses his/her words and hands to direct your attention to sensations of movement, often in ways that you last experienced in childhood. This refreshed image of yourself enables greater ease and precision in all actions.

AWARENESS THROUGH MOVEMENT®

A Feldenkrais Teacher verbally instructs an individual or group through gentle, sequenced movements, while asking questions which direct attention to differences in sensation. Participants learn at their own pace and in their own way, putting sensing and moving together to reduce unnecessary effort.

Founder

Moshe Feldenkrais, D.Sc. (1904 -1984), is world renowned for the system of body-awareness and exercises he developed during his lifetime. Moshe Feldenkrais studied engineering and went on to receive his doctorate in physics from the Sorbonne. While in Paris, he was attached to the lab of Joliot-Curie (Nobel Prize winner) and gained his Judo black belt with help from Professor Kano (creator of Judo). Over a period of 40 years, he synthesized his learning from mutiple disciplines into a method of somatic education that facilitates each student's ability to act efficiently and effectively.

P.S.

A Special Note from Ms. Louise

Although I had worked with many people before and after TKA surgery, I had never had the opportunity to see someone through every step of the process as outlined in this book.

Then, in the fall of 2013 when I was writing this book, I met a woman in her 60's who was scheduled for knee replacement surgery. She read the book and signed up to walk in Granny's shoes.

While the experience has been for her, as for others, challenging, the impact of her thorough preparation and the continuity of care, has been profound. From the astonished comments of hospital staff and family members, through her discovery that going through the lessons actually decreased her pain while improving her functional mobility, to her desire to spread the word.

It is with her blessing that I offer this road-tested gift to you.

—Louise Chegwidden, PT, FT
January 13, 2014

Without Whom...

NEAR ...

Martha Morris ~ the Matriarch of my neighborhood. Bless you, Granny.

Wendy Ellyn ~ for the lists and laughter and friendship ever after. I honor your keen eye and honest tongue, great gifts for an editor.

Paula Pagano and **Patrick Corkery** ~ your willingness to follow has led me for years.

Elaine Peterson ~ for your wisdom, courage, and endurance.

Peggy Kass ~ for your bright light and generous heart, and for spreading the word.

Anne Hightower ~ for your generous support both material and spiritual. Thank you for bounteous gifts, readily shared.

Leslie H. ~ for your impeccable timing and willingness to 'test-run' Ms. Linda's program. Your questions and trust changed the course of 'Granny' for the better.

Frank Wildman ~ for introducing me to Moshe's work, **Dennis Leri** and **Elizabeth Berringer** ~ for creating the conditions for learning, **Mia Segal** and **Leora Gaster** ~ for the joy, **Judith Dambowic** ~ for meticulous detailing assistance in the lessons, **Jeff Haller** ~ for reminding me to 'join the dots,' and every Feldenkrais teacher I've met ~ for the questions.

Mokhtar Paki ~ for giving the heart of the project visual life. What a pleasure to dance with you.

Alethea Walker and all the staff and councilors at Studio One ~ for providing a meeting place and resources for artists of all ages and persuasions.

Helen Krayenhoff ~ for advice—respectfully offered and gratefully received.

Claire Kiefer ~ for combing through the text with an eagle eye and for teaching me along the way.

Alvaro Villanueva ~ for converting the need for simplicity and accessibility into elegance.

Clients and **Students over the years** ~ my best teachers. Thank you for sharing your movement stories with me.

AND FAR

Lyn Small ~ for seeing the potential in an active 5 year old and following through with a lost teen. For making college possible and supporting my dreams. Thanks Mum.

Jennifer Back, Ann Hutton, and **Len Small** ~ for loving support over the long haul, *merci mille fois*.

ABOVE ...

Michael Chegwidden ~ for thinking the work I do in the world matters and for telling me so. For hugs to melt into. I miss you Dad.

Dr. Moshe Feldenkrais ~ for blazing a trail into the heart of whole body thinking. From the tips of my toes through my white and grey matter, my debt of gratitude is forever expanding.

Mark Reese ~ for embodying the power of 'less is more.' Your gentle, nuanced presence is fondly remembered.

AND BEYOND

My beloved son **Julian** ~ for constantly reminding me that if learning isn't fun, then it's work, and we just don't want to do it. Thank you for lending me the Gold Rush guys and introducing me to Mokhtar.

Cliff ~ my co-pilot in this wondrous life, and first eyes. 'Granny' is the richer for your mad wordcraft skills and insights. You make me laugh and bring me tea, who could ask for anything more?

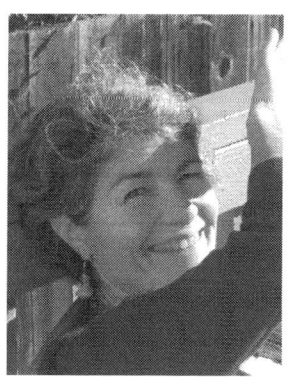

Louise Chegwidden was born in South Africa, grew up in Australia, and now resides in Oakland, California. The trajectory of her professional career as a Physical Therapist and Feldenkrais Teacher is remarkably similar to Ms. Linda's. She is an avid swimmer, commutes by bicycle, and loves to dance.

www.GrannyGetsANewKnee.com
www.LouiseChegwidden.com

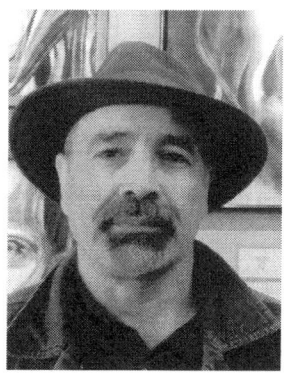

Mokhtar Paki was born in the Iranian city of Shiraz. He studied architecture in Iran and England before studying graphic design and lithography in Norway. He now lives in the San Francisco Bay Area, working as a visual artist, art teacher, author, and sometime architectural, set, and costume designer.

www.mokhtarimage.com

Made in the USA
Lexington, KY
08 April 2014